Comprehensive Care for H

A comprehensive health care system consists of services that are coordinated and integrated along the full continuum of care. For HIV patients, this includes physical health care, infectious disease management, crisis care, mental health care, substance abuse counseling, and social support services including housing, transportation, subsistence, and supports for dealing with multiple sources of stigma. This book highlights the dilemmas faced in delivering comprehensive, integrated care to individuals living with HIV, providing both an understanding of existing efforts to integrate diverse systems of care, as well as insight into ways in which systems of care must be challenged in order to meet the needs of people living with HIV. Comprehensive care for HIV/AIDS is the result of collaborative work with the county Health Department, numerous community-based organizations, and several planning boards in a metropolitan area, which have sought to provide integrated care to people living with HIV. It will be a valuable resource to the diverse community of HIV researchers, advocates, and providers.

Teresa L. Scheid is Professor of Sociology at the University of North Carolina at Charlotte, with appointments in Public Policy, Public Health, and Health Services Research.

Routledge Studies in Health and Social Welfare

Comprehensive Care for HIV/AIDS
Community-Based Strategies

Teresa L. Scheid

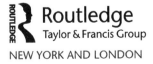
Routledge
Taylor & Francis Group

NEW YORK AND LONDON

First published 2015
by Routledge
711 Third Avenue, New York, NY 10017, USA

and by Routledge
2 Park Square, Milton Park, Abingdon, Oxfordshire OX14 4RN

First issued in paperback 2016

*Routledge is an imprint of the Taylor & Francis Group,
an informa business*

Library of Congress Cataloging-in-Publication Data

Scheid, Teresa L., author.
Comprehensive care for HIV/AIDS : community-based strategies / by
    Teresa L. Scheid.
        p. ; cm. — (Routledge studies in health and social welfare ; 12)
    Includes bibliographical references and index.
    I. Title.   II. Series: Routledge studies in health and social welfare ; 12.
[DNLM: 1. Community Health Services—organization &
administration.   2. HIV Infections.   3. Comprehensive Health
Care—organization & administration.   4. Continuity of Patient Care—
organization & administration. WC 503]
    RA643.8
    362.19697'92—dc23
    2014009885

Typeset in Sabon
by Apex CoVantage, LLC

ISBN 13: 978-1-138-28492-0 (pbk)
ISBN 13: 978-1-138-79178-7 (hbk)

Contents

Figures

Tables

Preface

An ideal health care system consists of services that are coordinated and integrated along the full continuum of care. For HIV/AIDS patients, this includes physical health care, infectious disease management, crisis care, mental health care, substance abuse counseling, and social support services including housing, transportation, subsistence, and supports for dealing with multiple sources of stigma. However, we do not have the conceptual tools or theoretical frameworks to direct these kinds of changes. In this volume, I highlight the dilemmas faced in providing comprehensive, integrated, wholistic care to individuals living with HIV disease. *Comprehensive Care for HIV/AIDS* provides both an understanding of existing efforts to integrate diverse systems of care, as well as insight into ways in which systems of care must be challenged in order to meet the needs of people living with HIV/AIDS.

This volume is the result of my collaborative work with the county Health Department, numerous community based organizations, and several community planning boards in the greater Charlotte region, which have sought in various ways to provide integrated care to people living with HIV/AIDS. I begin with client level data to highlight the negative synergy of living with multiple highly stigmatized health problems. I then turn to various ways in which the HIV/AIDS care system has sought to address these problems: case management, adherence counseling, and system wide cross training. Each chapter is based upon the efforts of providers to improve the system of HIV/AIDS care; however, these approaches are limited in that they do not address system wide sources of fragmentation. In the final two chapters, I address the work of three planning councils that developed comprehensive integration plans, describing how community planning can work and what factors work against efforts to reform systems of care.

The volume is an important addition to literature on HIV/AIDS care and service system integration, and will be of interest not only to HIV/AIDS providers, but to those who provide care to chronic care populations, and community health planners. Academically, it extends understanding of health care fragmentation and its ideological sources. It is also an important addition to the literature on community based participatory action research, as that framework is the basis for all the data collected. It is to this diverse community of clients, advocates, providers, and researchers that I address this volume.

I also want to thank those who I have worked so closely with the past 15 years. I began my work as a community researcher with Anne Dalton; together we moved from collaborative research in mental health to the HIV/AIDS Integration Project, and our efforts to integrate care continued on the HIV Task Force. Cheryl Emanual has been exemplary in her advocacy for improved community health and reducing health disparities. She has a remarkable ability to communicate and build consensus among diverse community stakeholders and I have learned so much from her. My co-collaborators in the numerous cross training projects described in Chapter 5 really stretched my teaching ability as I moved from the college classroom to the community—especially Joanne Jenkins, a goddess in every sense of the word. Finally, I want to thank Terry Ellington, who shares my over-riding concern with system level thinking and who continues to fight tirelessly to improve the HIV/AIDS system of care and collaboration.

1 Introduction

THE NATURE OF THE PROBLEM

We live in the midst of an epidemic, but not one that is widely acknowledged in the public realm. Nor has there been much academic analysis (Altman & Buse, 2014). New infections of HIV disease have remained relatively constant for several years, at around 40,000 each year, despite explicit goals set by the Centers for Disease Control (CDC) and numerous federal agencies to reduce the incidence of new cases of HIV. Data from the CDC show the number of new infections in 2010 was 47,129; and 33,015 were diagnosed with AIDS (CDC, 2012b). The National AIDS Strategy announced by President Obama in July 2010 (The White House, 2010) stated a commitment to reduce these rates by at least 25%. While new technologies may help us reach this goal (such as the use of HIV drugs to reduce the risk of contracting the virus, referred to as pre-exposure prophylaxis), reductions in funding for outreach and prevention may increase infections in the short run. Equally pressing, and the focus of this book, is the need to provide comprehensive care to those who are living with HIV disease. There are currently 1.2 million individuals living with HIV/AIDS (of whom 20% do not know they are infected) and in 2009, 17,774 people died of AIDS (CDC, 2012b).

The face of HIV/AIDS has changed during the past decade; rather than a disease found primarily among gay, White men, it is now a health crisis in minority communities. In fact, HIV disease meets the conditions of a generalized epidemic where prevalence rates exceed 1% (and rates are much higher among African Americans); both the CDC and academic researchers refer to HIV as an epidemic (CDC, 2012b; Pellowski, Kalichman, Lews, & Adler, 2013). As has been well documented, Blacks and Hispanics are at higher risk for new infections of HIV. While Blacks constituted only 14% of the population in 2009, they accounted for 44% of new HIV/AIDS diagnoses in the U.S., and in 2008 they accounted for 46% or people living with HIV and Hispanics accounted for 20% of new HIV cases (CDC, 2012b).[1] Among Blacks, women are at growing risk for HIV infection; the rate of new HIV cases for Black women is 15 times that of White women and three times that of Hispanic women (CDC, 2012b). Furthermore, African

Americans continue to have the highest age-adjusted death rate due to HIV disease. In 2007, HIV was the ninth cause of death for Blacks and the third leading cause of death for Blacks aged 34–44 (CDC, 2012a). The public misconception is that injection drug use is the primary factor behind the HIV crisis, especially in the Black community, but in this regard the face of HIV disease is similar to that of HIV disease worldwide: risky sexual contact. In 2006, heterosexual transmission accounted for 31% of new cases, while new infections due to injection drug use was only 12%—down 80% (Kaiser Family Foundation [KFF], 2013a). The primary transmission category for Black men living with HIV disease is sexual contact with men, followed by injection drug use. For Black women the primary transmission route is high risk heterosexual contact (CDC, 2012a).

Socioeconomic conditions certainly play a fundamental role in both the higher rates of HIV infection for African Americans and the lower rates of treatment leading to higher rates of death at younger ages. Nearly 1 in 4 Blacks live in poverty, and many more than that face significant barriers to adequate health care, including a lack of minority or culturally competent health care providers. Minority groups report significant barriers to care (Phillip, Mayer, & Aday, 2000), in large part due to a lack of cultural accessibility. Anderson (2000), in analysis of a national probability sample of those in treatment for HIV, found that vulnerable groups (i.e., women, injection drug users, African Americans, and those with lower educational levels) were least likely to gain early access to antiretroviral medications. The National Health Disparities Report also reviews evidence showing that African American's are less likely to receive standard HIV care (as cited in Pellowski et al., 2013). African Americans with a White health provider experienced longer delays between diagnosis and treatment than when their health provider is also Black (Earnshaw, Bogard, Dovidio, & Williams, 2013). Disparities in medical treatment further exacerbate disparities in incidence and access to care in minorities communities.

Individuals with a positive HIV diagnosis are also at risk for mental health problems (Batki, 1990; Crystal & Schlosser, 1999; Simoni & Ng, 2000). In addition to anxiety and depression following a positive HIV diagnosis, HIV seropositivity strains social relationships and supports, and results in a great deal of stress due to concern over work status and the experience of ongoing illnesses, as well as adherence to complicated drug regimes. Results from the Steps study of individuals newly diagnosed with HIV show that 67% of respondents were depressed (Bhatia, Hartman, Kallen, Graham, & Giordano, 2011). Depression may be even higher for those HIV-positive individuals with substance abuse problems (Berger-Greenstein et al., 2007). For these reasons, assessment and treatment plans for individuals with HIV/AIDS need to include a comprehensive biopsychosocial assessment (Rubenstein & Sorrentino, 2008).

Poverty is an important factor in considering the status of those living with HIV, regardless of race. Pellowski et al. (2013, p. 205) argue that

"HIV infection is so closely enmeshed in conditions of poverty that it is indeed a pandemic of the poor." Conover, Arno, Weaver, Ang, and Ettner (2006) report that more than half of those with HIV, mental health, and substance abuse diagnoses lived below the poverty line, and the majority of their income came from public sources. The HIV/AIDS Treatment Adherence, Health Outcomes and Cost Study has examined the issues surrounding health care access and costs for care for individuals diagnosed with HIV/AIDS, mental health, and substance abuse problems (Conover, Weaver, Ang, Arno, Flynn, & Ettner, 2009). These authors report baseline expenditures of $3,880 per month. Consequently, individuals living with HIV often have to rely on public assistance to pay their medical costs (Conover, Weaver, Arno, Ang, & Ettner, 2010), which certainly raises important policy issues about how such care will continue to be paid for.

There is a need for continuity of care and a comprehensive array of services for those living with HIV, and mental health and substance abuse problems. However, HIV disease, substance abuse, and mental health services are delivered within independent service systems and organizations (Meyerson & Scofield, 1999). Providers generally have expertise in one, perhaps two, areas of disability and illness—HIV/AIDS, mental health, or substance abuse. Because of the co-occurrence of mental illness and substance abuse, many mental health care providers do have training in substance abuse, although treatment orientations differ (Burton, Cox, & Fleisher-Bond, 2001). Mental health and substance abuse providers often lack basic training in HIV disease and are unsure how to assess a client's risk. HIV providers may have some background in either substance abuse or mental health, but may not be able to recognize or deal effectively with a client's substance abuse or mental health problems. Because of heavy caseloads and multiple demands, providers often work in isolation and have limited connections to other types of treatment providers and services.

Currently, health care researchers use the term "co-morbid" (or co-occurring) to refer to individuals with multiple physical and mental health problems. The term "co-morbid" arose from literature addressing chronic or serious mental illness, and co-morbid substance abuse problems. It was extended to include individuals who are HIV-positive and also have substance abuse problems, and there is a great deal of literature on both of these treatment populations, as they have been the focus of sustained governmental funding and research. Generally, co-morbidity has been limited to understandings of two highly co-morbid conditions that have negative impacts on one another (such as mental health and substance abuse [SA], or HIV and SA). The idea of co-morbidity is theoretically based on that of intersectionality—individuals have characteristics which intersect, or overlap, one another.[2] However, as Figure 1.1 illustrates, the idea of co-morbidity or intersectionality does not fully capture the complexity groups with multiple problems face.

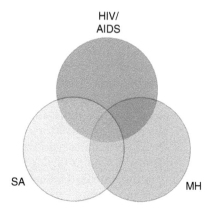

Figure 1.1   Co-Morbidity

Sociologists have used the concept of "cumulative disadvantage" to capture the idea that poverty and racism have strong multiplicative effects (DiPrete & Eirich, 2006). The idea of cumulative disadvantage is illustrated in Figure 1.2. However, this concept fails to capture the truly synergistic interaction between HIV, mental health, and substance abuse within populations experiencing poverty and racism, as well as multiple sources of stigma. As defined by the *Merriam-Webster Dictionary*, synergies produce effects of which each part is individually incapable. Similar to the sociological concept of organicism, the whole cannot be reduced to its parts. However, the concept of synergy is misleading because it implies a kind of energy, when, in fact, individuals facing multiple health problems within the context of poverty, racism, and stigma experience a downward pull, or negative synergy. When faced with multiple sources of stigma, as well as debilitating illnesses, one's self-concept is seriously undermined. Stigma also results in social isolation and loss of social supports (Pellowski et al., 2013). Add to the stress of illness and poverty, the loss of social supports and personal coping mechanisms, and you have a group that will be extremely difficult to treat. Without major structural changes to existing social systems (such as eliminating poverty, racism, and stigma), the only route out of the downward spiral is for individuals to develop stronger coping mechanisms and social support networks to help them deal with the stress of their illnesses. Consequently, both clinical and research efforts have been directed at the individual, rather than the structural level.

Ask any HIV, mental health (MH), or SA clients about their health care providers and they will generally mention one person who has provided them with crucial social support, as well as treatment. Often these individuals are case managers who assist clients to meet their basic needs. Yet, health care providers are trained and operate within distinct service sectors (HIV, MH, or SA) and are poorly equipped to deal with the "secondary" problems of poverty, racism, and stigma. While the necessity of multidisciplinary

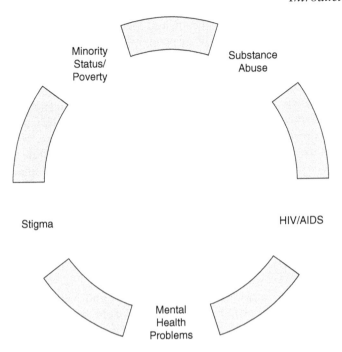

Figure 1.2   Cumulative Disadvantage

treatment teams and cross-training has been recognized, these mechanisms fall short of achieving the ideal goal of integrated care. Providers do engage in advocacy, but these efforts are generally directed toward the individual client rather than toward the system of care. Governmental agencies, such as the Centers for Disease Control and Substance Abuse and Mental Health Services Administration (SAMHSA), advocate integrated systems of care for individuals living with HIV and other co-morbid conditions. However, the principles articulated by these agencies are based on a medicalized, individualized approach to the problem of living with HIV disease, and actually work against system integration. As illustrated in Figure 1.1 with co-morbidity, the multiple problems faced by people living with HIV/AIDS are treated in a categorical way, in large part due to separate funding streams. I next provide background on how HIV care is currently funded, as funding is the driver behind service provision and systems of care.

FUNDING FOR HIV CARE

I focus on public sector funding for HIV rather than private insurance. This is because the majority of people living with HIV are poor; nearly half live on less than $10,000 a year, and most of those living with HIV disease lack insurance (Conover et al., 2009). There are three sources of public funding for HIV care: Ryan White, Medicaid, and Medicare. Medicaid is the largest source of funding, covering half of people with HIV in regular care (KFF, 2013b). The Affordable Care Act has just been recently implemented (October 2013) and will affect how many individuals are eligible for Medicaid (in those states that have accepted Medicaid expansion) and able to negotiate finding their own health insurance via the state and federal exchanges or the insurance marketplace. In those states that have accepted the federal expansion of Medicaid, there will be increased access to HIV care. North Carolina (the state within which data for this book has been collected) joined a majority of southern states that refused the Medicaid expansion and are not running their own exchange. Without the Medicaid expansion, a large number of individuals living with HIV will still be denied health care coverage in North Carolina. These individuals will no doubt continue to deteriorate, and will ultimately cost the health care system more than if they were able to receive treatment at an earlier stage of illness. At this time, there is a great deal of uncertainty about both the short- and long-term impacts of the Affordable Care Act on HIV disease.

Medicaid is the largest source of HIV funds and provides coverage to an estimated 230,000 people living with HIV, approximately 1 in 4 people living with HIV (KFF, 2013b). Individuals living in poverty and who are permanently disabled receive Medicaid. Individuals living with HIV who are over 65 are also eligible for Medicare, and approximately 20% of those receiving HIV care are covered by Medicare (KFF, 2013b). Approximately 25% of Medicaid beneficiaries with HIV are dually eligible for both Medicaid and Medicare, and their drug costs are paid for by Medicare under Part D, while other health care costs are paid for by Medicaid. Unlike Medicare (which is funded solely by the federal government), Medicaid is jointly funded by the federal government and states, leading to a great deal of variability in funding. However, states must provide inpatient and outpatient services, physician and laboratory services, and long-term care. Optional services include prescription drug services and many other health care services, such as dental care, psychosocial rehabilitation, and case management.

Ryan White is the largest federal program designed specifically for people living with HIV. The Ryan White Comprehensive AIDS Resources Emergency (CARE) Act was passed in 1990 following the death of Ryan White, a young White boy with hemophilia who experienced discrimination and ostracism due to his HIV status. The Ryan White CARE Act provides funding for HIV care, education, and prevention, and funding must be re-appropriated by Congress every year. Ryan White was designed to be the payor of last resort, and continues to fill gaps not covered by other sources of funding (both public and private). The Ryan White CARE Act has been reauthorized four times (most recently in 2009), and its focus changed significantly in the 2006 re-authorization. At that time, funding was shifted toward core medical services. Before I explain what this means for HIV care and prevention services, I will provide a bit more on the organization of the Ryan White Program.

While administrated by the Health Resources and Services Administration (HRSA) of the U.S. Department of Health and Human Services, Ryan White funding provides for significant state and local control of HIV planning and service delivery. Community based organizations (CBOs) constitute close to half of those serving clients with Ryan White dollars (KFF, 2009), and CBOs include multi-agency consortiums whose formation was initiated and has been supported by Ryan White dollars (Lune, 2007). Ryan White is divided into different Parts—Part A to Part F. Part A (which constitutes 20% of the Ryan White dollars) provides money to Eligible Metropolitan Areas (EMAs) and Transitional Grant Areas (TGAs) whose cumulative totals for AIDS exceed 2,000 EMAs or are in the range of 1,000–1,900 TGAs. Charlotte, North Carolina, qualified as a TGA in 2006 after the reauthorization. Part B has the largest share of Ryan White funding (55%) and provides support, including funds for patient drug assistance programs, to all 50 states, the District of Columbia, Puerto Rico, Guam, the U.S. Virgin Islands, and all five territories (KFF, 2009). Funding is for direct service provision and can be accessed directly (most often by health departments) or by Part B "Consortia," which are associations authorized by the original Ryan White to plan for and deliver services (much of my work has been in collaboration with the Regional HIV/AIDS Consortium in Charlotte, NC). Part C (9%) provides for early intervention services, Part D (3%) is for family and community based services, and Part F (4%) provides funding for AIDS Education and Training Centers, Dental Programs, the Minority AIDS Initiative, and Special Projects of National Significance.

Ryan White also provides money for the AIDS Drug Assistance Program (ADAP), which is administered by the states under Part B. As HIV care increasingly revolves around adherence to complicated anti-retroviral drug regimes, which are very costly (see Chapter 4), the 2006 reauthorization emphasized the provision of designated "core medical services." Seventy-five percent of funding for Parts A to C (93% of total Ryan White dollars) must be spent on what have been defined as core medical services: ambulatory and outpatient medical care, medications, early intervention, home health care, medical nutrition therapy, hospice, home and community based services, mental health and substance abuse outpatient care, and medical case management. The other 25% can pay for what are deemed support services: food banks, emergency housing assistance, legal services, various forms of psychosocial support, medical transportation, outreach, and emergency financial assistance. The Ryan White reauthorization constitutes a "medicalization" of HIV care—a theme that runs through this book and that I analyze more fully in the concluding chapter. At this point, it is suffice to say funding restrictions by Ryan White (and most recently, Medicaid) have served to change the types of services available to HIV clients, with increasing emphasis on an individualized, medical symptom-based treatment that mitigates against the kinds of comprehensive, integrated systems of care that allow for wholistic care. This book details the experiences of one urban community that has received funding and maintains a sustained goal of providing for coordinated comprehensive care, demonstrating what can be done, identifying barriers to integrated systems of care, and developing programs to improve systems of care.

SOURCES OF DATA AND INSIGHT

The majority of the data utilized in this book came from clients and providers in Mecklenburg County, North Carolina. Mecklenburg County has very high rates of HIV disease, accounting for 20% of new cases reported in North Carolina. Between 1999 and 2008, HIV case rates (the number of HIV-positive individuals per 100,000) increased by 57%. Case rates were even higher in 2008 (55.9), but slowed to 34.1 in 2010, with a slight increase in 2011 (NC HIV/AIDS database, data obtained from the Mecklenburg County Health Department). Hardest hit have been African Americans, who represent over 70% of the new cases, despite being only 30% of the county's population. HIV infections among Hispanics have also increased. As a result of the high HIV case rates, in 2007, Mecklenburg County and the surrounding five counties in the Standard Metropolitan Statistical Area were designated as a Transitional Grant Area (TGA) by the Ryan White HIV/AIDS Treatment Authorization Act. As a TGA, Mecklenburg County is defined by the federal government to be "severely and disproportionately affected by HIV disease." As of December 31, 2011, there were 4,715 individuals living with HIV disease in Mecklenburg County (North Carolina HIV/STD Surveillance Report, 2011). However, the CDC estimates that as many as 21% of persons with HIV are unaware of their status; consequently, there are at least another thousand individuals living with HIV disease in the county who are unaware of their status.

Mecklenburg County is also unique in the number of HIV-positive individuals who are on wait lists for HIV medications. The AIDS Drug Assistance Program (ADAP) under Ryan White provides for lifesaving HIV medications, but state dollars are matched by federal dollars. Only 10 states routinely have wait lists for HIV medications. North Carolina is one of those states, and Mecklenburg County routinely has the highest number on the wait list in the state. Luckily, in August 2012, the Department of Health and Human Services (in response to advocacy efforts) released 75 million dollars in emergency funding for HIV medications, temporarily reducing wait lists. However, it is expected that problems funding ADAP will remain as the state moves further into a fiscal crisis engendered by the recession. More critically, those states that opted out of the Medicaid expansion will not get federal matching funds. Data reported by the National ADAP Monitoring Project Annual Report, 2012, show that North Carolina had experienced a 26%

decline in funding for ADAP, perhaps in response to increased federal funding (www.nastad.org). The future is most uncertain for the close to 7,000 individuals currently enrolled in ADAP in North Carolina.

While I can make no claims to the generalizability of these data, clearly, as a case study, Mecklenburg County and surrounding counties in the Standard Metropolitan Statistical Area (SMSA) of Charlotte, North Carolina, offer providers and advocates with important insights on the need for, and paths to, comprehensive systems of care for those living with HIV disease. This book is the result of my collaborative work with various community agencies in the greater Charlotte region that have sought to provide integrated care to people living with HIV. I first worked with the county health department to secure funding for cross-training for providers working in HIV, MH, and SA. Ultimately, the health department obtained Substance Abuse and Mental Health Services Administration (SAMHSA) funding for a planning grant to integrate services for minority populations at risk for HIV/AIDS with co-occurring mental health and substance abuse problems (this language reflects the granting agency's perspective of the problem). I was the formative evaluator on the grant, which provided support for a 2-year planning process (2000–2002) and mandated the active involvement of providers, as well as consumers, in the development of an integration plan.

As the formative evaluator, I played a critical role in the development of the plan, which required developing a broad based consensus among a number of diverse groups, organizations, and individuals. The process and the integration plan we developed is described in Chapter 6. While financial support for the integration plan did not materialize, the core group of participants continued to meet and, in 2004, we were officially recognized as the HIV Task Force and asked by the County Commissioners to develop a plan to address the problems of HIV disease.

I had officially become an advocate, and found myself taking a leadership role in the development of consensus behind a plan that would have a fairly immediate impact (and it did, the County Commissioners provided over $300,000 in additional monies for HIV care to the health department). I continue to play an active role and am currently the secretary and organization driver for what is now called the HIV/AIDS Council, which meets on a monthly basis and continues to work to improve systems of care for individuals living with HIV disease.

My role in the community has provided me with numerous opportunities to collect data, not only in terms of my own participation on various planning boards, but as an extension of my research role on several key grants.[3] Agency efforts to secure funding led to the Regional HIV/AIDS Consortium (which had served a 13-county area) gaining an enhanced substance abuse treatment grant (2002–2007) from the SAMHSA. I served as the evaluator on that grant, and collected data from clients referred to the program. SAMHSA provided an initial data tracking instrument that we augmented to include additional areas of concern (such as adherence and social support).

Staff at the Consortium completed the relatively short instrument with clients referred to the program at intake, and at 6-month and 12-month follow up points. Over the course of the 5-year grant, intake data was collected on 320 clients, 6-month follow up data on 229 clients, and 12-month follow up data on 176 clients. While the focus of the grant was on enhanced substance abuse services, we collected data on mental health problems, as well.

I also collected in-depth data from 40 clients who called me voluntarily in the first 2 years of the grant and completed a telephone interview for $10. This interview contained open-ended questions based on Arthur Kleinman's Illness Narratives (1988), as well as questions about relations with health care providers, substance abuse, and adherence. In addition, fixed choice questions were included to assess self-esteem, hope, relations with providers, and social support. Both sets of client-level data are used in Chapter 2 to illustrate the mental health needs of people living with HIV disease.

In addition, I have collected fairly extensive data from providers—primarily case managers. The SAMHSA enhanced substance abuse project mandated four meetings per year with case managers and substance abuse providers, and I surveyed these providers at the spring meeting annually. The data collected from providers assessed not only information about the needs of providers' patients, but also their own training needs, emotional labor, burnout, and sources of job satisfaction and dissatisfaction, as well as an understanding of diverse systems of care and cultural competency. These data will be utilized in Chapter 3 to understand how case managers approach the problems of clients with HIV and the barriers they face in their work.

A fairly rich source of data that links clients and providers resulted from my role in developing procedures for adherence counseling. The Regional HIV/AIDS Consortium obtained a private grant that funded three specialized adherence counselors. None of the three providers had previous experience in adherence, and we worked together for 3 months to develop an in-depth understanding of adherence, as well as creating instruments that served both clinical and research purposes. Over 50 clients were referred for adherence counseling, and in-depth data was collected from each client. In addition to monthly meetings, the three adherence counselors completed 3-month progress notes on each client. Ultimately, we developed an adherence manual that was used in training various groups of providers (primarily HIV case managers) to "do adherence." While adherence has generated an overwhelming number of studies, it has been primarily understood as a medical problem to be solved on the individual level (Farmer, 2005). The problem of adherence serves as an exemplar for the medicalized thinking about HIV, which has driven current funding sources and ultimately systems (or non-systems) of care—a theme I develop throughout the book.

I also served as a member of the interdisciplinary cross-training team. This group started in 1996 as a result of providers' own recognition of the need for cross-training in order to deal with the multiple needs of their

HIV clients. A group of about 10 dedicated individuals meet monthly and derived an experiential cross-training curriculum, which various agencies (the Health Department, Regional Consortium, and Area Health Education Center) funded. This group was the original purpose for my working with the health department and securing the SAMHSA integration grant. However, I became a faculty member and worked to modify cross-trainings and conduct them over the course of several years, and also wrote two National Institutes of Health grant proposals to more systematically evaluate the effectiveness of experiential as opposed to didactic cross-trainings. I also worked with the SAMHSA's cross-training modules in the course of the enhanced substance abuse treatment grant, and ultimately collected data on the effectiveness of cross-training. This data is used in Chapter 5 to describe how cross-training can advance collaboration between providers and consumers, and also points to the limits of cross-training in developing integrated systems of care.

The majority of the data collected and used in this book was based on the principles of community based participatory action research (CBPR). CBPR is not a method, but an orientation to research (Minkler & Wallerstein, 2003) that involves collaborative research targeting locally defined issues, often with the goal of eliminating health disparities (Farquhar, Michael, & Wiggens, 2005). The "community" is defined both geographically (providers, advocates, and consumers in the Charlotte SMSA and Mecklenburg County) and by a common identity. As described above, there has been a long history of voluntary involvement by providers, advocates, and consumers in finding ways to improve the HIV service system, especially for minority communities. There have been literally thousands of hours spent by individuals coming together on their own time to meet and collect data and develop strategies to integrate care. We worked together to develop protocols for the provision of care, which also provided us with needed data for either the development of grants to fund these services, or to use in advocacy efforts to increase local funding for services. In addition to collaboration between academic researchers and the community, CBPR aims to develop knowledge that can be disseminated to other communities. The book combines data on services and provider based techniques (e.g., principles for adherence counseling and cross-training curriculum), which will be useful for those seeking to understand HIV care and the work of HIV care providers, researchers, and community planners.

OVERVIEW OF THE BOOK

As articulated by Shortell, Giles, and Anderson (2000), an ideal health care system consists of services that are coordinated and integrated along the full continuum of care. For HIV patients, this includes physical health care, infectious disease management, crisis care, mental health care, substance abuse counseling, and social support services including housing, transportation, subsistence, and supports for dealing with multiple sources of stigma. However, we do not have the conceptual tools or theoretical frameworks to direct these kinds of changes. In this book, I highlight the dilemmas faced in providing comprehensive, integrated, wholistic care to individuals living with HIV disease. This book provides both an understanding of existing efforts to integrate diverse systems of care, and insight into ways in which systems of care must be challenged in order to meet the needs of people with HIV.

I begin in Chapter 2 with those who are living with HIV to highlight the negative synergy of living with multiple highly stigmatized health problems. Combined with poverty and minority status, people with HIV live in a state of elevated stress, exacerbating all too normal feelings of depression and anxiety. I use both qualitative and quantitative data to examine the sources and consequences of mental health problems among individuals living with HIV who had been referred to the aforementioned enhanced substance abuse project. Social supports are critical, and I end Chapter 2 with a consideration of peer based social supports, and the importance of these types of groups for consumer advocacy.

A critical source of social support for individuals living with HIV disease is their health care providers. In Chapter 3, I use data collected from case managers, counselors, and nurses who provide care to HIV-positive individuals to examine not only their understanding of the complex nature of their clients' problems and their treatment ideologies, but the barriers they face in providing comprehensive care. Chapter 4 extends our understanding of the work of case managers and counselors by focusing on the work of three adherence counselors who were funded for 3 years to improve the treatment adherence of clients referred to them. Chapter 4 describes how practitioners and researchers can work together to both improve clinical care and develop procedures for the dissemination of that information. The Adherence Project is a good example of community based participatory research. Both Chapters 3 and 4 conclude with a consideration as to how changes in Ryan White and Medicaid funding for case management have changed the role of case managers, and have undermined the social support functions traditionally filled by case managers.

Chapter 5 focuses on cross-training—the principle tool used to provide integrated care to clients with HIV disease and co-occurring MH and SA problems. I introduce an experiential model developed and refined by a core faculty working together for close to 10 years to provide cross-training. This model is not a set curriculum, as it involves a number of strategies to enhance active learning, but it does provide a framework for diverse communities to design their own cross-training modules. The chapter focuses on both the need for and advantages of cross-training, as well as its limitations.

In Chapter 6, I return to the larger topic of system integration. I provide a more detailed discussion of the subject, and review of approaches to achieve system integration for individuals living with HIV, SA, and MH problems. The experience and results of an intensive integration planning project (funded by SAMHSA) are described, with the purpose to demonstrate how community planning can work, and what factors will work against implementation of efforts to reform systems of care. I describe how local HIV advocates have continued to work to achieve a better, more integrated system of HIV care via more direct political involvement with the local government through the formation of an HIV Task Force, which has ultimately become formally recognized as the Mecklenburg County HIV/AIDS Council. Once again, the barriers to system integration are highlighted.

Chapter 7 serves as a conclusion and points to the opportunities for enhanced advocacy that limited funding opens up. I begin by describing a very successful World AIDS Day 2010 in Charlotte, North Carolina—the first time a broad based coalition worked together to plan a public event with culmination being reading of a public HIV proclamation by one of the County Commissioners. While individual agencies and community based organizations (CBOs) have not been able to advocate directly for their clients, coalitions of consumers and providers can. I also describe the unique problems faced by researchers who find themselves working with groups as advocates; a critical issue for community based participatory researchers. I then turn to a more theoretical consideration of system fragmentation—focusing on categorical approaches to illness, and individualized, medicalized approaches to care, which exacerbate domain disputes between organizations serving clients with multiple health care needs. I conclude by presenting a model for wholistic care, which moves beyond the models for co-morbidity and cumulative disadvantage presented in this chapter. This framework can provide advocates, providers, and consumers with some wider understanding of how to change and improve systems of HIV care.

NOTES

1. The Centers for Disease Control and the Kaiser Family Foundation (KFF) are both good sources for updated information on the epidemiology of HIV/AIDS. As of this writing (2013), both sources were using 2010 data on prevalence and new transmissions.
2. Intersectionality has also been used to refer to the intersection of multiple minority statuses: gender, race, sexual orientation, and social class; and is an important perspective for those studying health disparities (Bowleg, 2012). I return to an enhanced discussion of this broader use of the term intersectionality in the concluding chapter.
3. All forms of data collection were approved by the UNC-Charlotte Institutional Review Board.

2 Living with HIV Disease
Mental Health, Substance Use, and Social Supports

INTRODUCTION

This chapter examines the experience of living with HIV disease, focusing on the multiple problems experienced by individuals living with HIV. I utilize client-level data collected between 2002 and 2007 by the Regional HIV/AIDS Consortium (serving a 13-county area and headquartered in Charlotte, North Carolina). The project was funded by the Substance Abuse and Mental Health Services Administration (SAMSHA) and was one of over 250 targeted capacity grants for enhanced substance abuse services. I served as the evaluator on the project. Each year, a maximum of 68 clients were referred to enhanced substance abuse services (referrals were generally made by case managers), and each client was interviewed at in-take, 6 months, and 12 months by staff at the Regional HIV/AIDS Consortium. The same individual interviewed the clients for all three interviews and worked to get the client into substance abuse treatment, hence playing the role of a clinician researcher. The instrument used was developed by SAMHSA, and was enhanced by me to collect additional data on social support and treatment adherence. While the data was entered in a governmental data tracking system, I also entered the data into my own software program for analysis. Over the course of the 5-year grant, intake data was collected on 320 clients, 6-month follow up data on 229 clients, and 12-month follow up data on 176 clients.

I also interviewed 43 clients who were part of the larger enhanced substance abuse project. This interview contained open-ended questions based on Arthur Kleinman's Illness Narratives (see Appendix A) about relations with health care providers, substance abuse, and adherence. Both these sets of client-level data will be used in this chapter to illustrate the multiple needs of people living with HIV disease. The qualitative data is used to explore the experience of living with HIV disease, stigma, and mental health problems associated with living with HIV disease, and the importance of social supports. While there are many good qualitative studies of individuals living with HIV disease (Baumgartner, 2007; Gentry, 2007; Trainor & Ezer, 2000; Whetton-Goldstein & Nguyen, 2002), the data presented in this chapter allows the voices of those who are the ultimate beneficiaries of the integration strategies developed to be heard. The Kleinman Illness Narratives allow individuals to describe their illness in their own terms, and hence provides insight into their health beliefs, which are critical to understanding barriers to care. The quantitative data provides a more systematic analysis of those factors associated with substance use and mental health problems among those living with HIV. I begin with a brief overview of the co-occurrence of HIV, mental health, and substance abuse, and the role of social support. I conclude this chapter with a discussion of the role of peer based social supports in enhancing behavioral health outcomes.

LIVING WITH HIV: DEPRESSION, SUBSTANCE USE, AND SOCIAL SUPPORTS

Individuals with a positive HIV diagnosis are at higher risk for mental health problems. Depression is a normal reaction to any chronic illness, but is especially likely with a positive HIV diagnosis (Batki, 1990; Crystal & Schlosser, 1999; Simoni & Ng, 2000). Living with HIV disease is also a significant source of ongoing stress and can exacerbate normal feelings of depression and anxiety. Individuals who are HIV-positive experience poor physical health; consequently, many face disruptions in work status and income. HIV disease is highly stigmatizing and often results in the loss of social support systems and networks (Whetten-Goldstein & Nguyen, 2002). The loss of social supports and outright discrimination and ostracism can exacerbate depression, anxiety, and suicidal ideation.

Researchers have consistently found elevated rates of mental health disorders among HIV patients. Komiti et al. (2003) found 22% of 322 HIV patients in general practice had major depressive disorder. In a study of 180 individuals newly diagnosed with HIV, Bhatia, Hartman, Kallen, Graham, and Giordano (2011) found that 67% were depressed. Other researchers have also found that HIV clients have high rates of depression (Berger-Greenstein et al., 2007), mental illness (Pence et al., 2005), and symptoms of mental health problems (Whetten et al., 2005). Women have higher rates of depression than men (Wisniewski et al., 2005), and minority status is also associated with higher risk for mental health problems (Winiarski et al., 2005). However, all too often mental health services are lacking for people living with HIV. In a recent survey of 2,052 HIV-positive people (the survey was conducted jointly by AIDSmeds, POZ, the National Association of People with AIDS, and the American Psychological Association in 2008), only 4% had not experienced some kind of psychological problem since their HIV diagnosis. Three fourths (1,500) had tried to discuss their mental health problems with their primary health care provider, but close to one third (28%) were not referred to mental health care. Of those who did receive mental health counseling, 30% were not satisfied with that counseling, the most common reason being that mental health providers were not familiar with the problems caused by HIV disease (www.poz.com/articles/hiv_apa_survey_401_16526.shtml).

Substance abuse is also commonly associated with HIV—not just as a cause (Klinkenberg & Sacks, 2004), but as a consequence because individuals self-medicate and may use substances as an escape. Drug use can increase the physical effects of HIV disease and increase illness burden (Tsao, Dobalian, & Stein, 2005), and can also exacerbate emotional distress in HIV-positive individuals (Komiti et al., 2003; Nnadi, Better, Take, Herning, & Cadet, 2002). Depression and mental health problems have also been found to be associated with poor treatment adherence (Catz, Kelly, Bogard, Benotsch, & McAuliffe, 2000; Cook et al., 2002; Murphy, Marelich, Hoffman, & Steers, 2004; Tucker, Burnam, Sherbourne, Kung, & Gifford 2003).

Social support has been associated with both physical and mental health outcomes, and has been widely studied across a number of disciplines. Social support has been linked to improved health outcomes for individuals living with HIV disease (Burgoyne & Renwick, 2004; Gielen, McDonnell, Wu, O'Campo, & Faden, 2001; Jia et al., 2004; Stewart, Cianfrini, & Walker, 2005). Social support has also been associated with improved mental health outcomes (or lower levels of depression and distress) for those living with HIV disease (Komiti et al., 2003; Silver, Bauman, Camacho, & Hudis, 2003). Reich, Lounsbury, Zaid-Muhammad, and Rapkin (2010) found that social support from someone important to the respondent was more strongly associated with positive mental health than having only general support and assistance.

Social support has been found to have a positive effect on adherence (Broadhead et al., 2002; Catz et al., 2000; Power et al., 2003). Good social support systems can help individuals deal with complicated medication regimes and also signal acceptance of the illness, which can lead not only to adherence, but to enhanced self-esteem and lower levels of emotional distress. Silver, Bauman, Camacho, and Hudis (2003) found that psychological distress was exacerbated by a lack of adequate social support. Having a significant other (i.e., partner) was found to lower the odds of depression among HIV clients in general practice (Komiti et al., 2003). Jai et al. (2004) found that social support and coping resources decreased depression and led to higher levels of health related quality of life. They conclude that more strategies are needed for improving social supports and coping resources for individuals living with HIV disease. However, the type of social support provided must match the type of stressor. Thoits (2011, p. 151) has distinguished between social support from primary ties and secondary ties, finding that secondary ties may be a more important source of social support when an individual is faced with "acute negative stressors and intensified ongoing strains" (such as living with HIV). Family and friends (primary others) may exacerbate the stress of HIV because of the stigma associated with the disease and the resources needed to provide ongoing support to one living with a chronic disease. More positive supports may be offered by secondary social relationships, such as other HIV-positive individuals, health care providers, or other community groups.

While most providers are aware their clients face a great deal of stigma, they do not have a full understanding of how stigma operates, nor do they fully appreciate how formidable a barrier stigma is to clients' acceptance of their illness and to the availability of social supports. Stigma leads to poorer mental health and physical health outcomes, and a loss of social supports (Pellowski et al., 2013). Parker and Aggleton (2003) argue that the reason HIV stigma is so persistent is the source of the stigma lies in socioeconomic power structures. As noted by Link and Phelan (2001, p. 375) "it takes power to stigmatize." However, providers tend to see stigma as residing at the individual level, and focus on the need for enhanced personal coping mechanisms. Addressing stigma at the structural level involves dealing with structural sources of health disparities, such as residential segregation and the chronic stress of both poverty and discrimination faced by minorities (Earnshaw et al., 2013).

Providers are also more likely to use individually based approaches to treatment and prevention, relying on behavioral models that focus on motivation and self-efficacy (Prado, Lightfoot, & Brown, 2013). A substance abuse counselor would seek to deal with the substance abuse first, then HIV meds, then seek mental health counseling. Solutions are sought for separate, individual problems within a medical model, and do not adequately address the complexity of the negative synergy that results from multiple health problems that are highly stigmatized. Gender, race, and sexuality intersect in complex ways for individuals living with HIV, leading to increased stigma and lowered self-efficacy, as well as higher levels of psychological distress (Prado et al., 2013).

The qualitative data I collected from HIV clients provides some insight into how the complexities of living with HIV disease are experienced by individuals. Many individuals are in denial about their illness, fearful to even give it a name, itself a critical barrier to health care. Feelings of isolation, loneliness, and depression were common—emotions that can exacerbate the physical effects of HIV. Critical to living with HIV disease was supportive relationships.

THE LIVED EXPERIENCE OF HIV DISEASE

I conducted in-depth telephone interviews with 43 clients who had been referred to the SAMHSA enhanced substance abuse services project. My goal was to arrive at greater understanding of how clients experience their illness. A notice was distributed by case managers and Consortium staff during the first 2 years of the study (2000–2002) that asked clients to call my toll free number to "participate in a confidential research study about coping with HIV/AIDS." The flyer targeted problems with HIV medications, problems caused by HIV/AIDS, or "what could be done to help people with HIV/AIDS." Potential respondents were advised the interview would take 15 to 20 minutes, and they would be reimbursed $10 for their participation. They were instructed to leave a number and time they could be reached, but to not leave their name. Conditions for the informed consent was listed on the notice and read by either case managers or Consortium staff (the interview protocol was approved by the UNC-Charlotte Institutional Review Board). Despite IRB concerns over anonymity, most respondents left their name and had no qualms with my mailing the $10 to their homes or the homes of friends/family members. I, unfortunately, have no way to track response bias, but the respondents were demographically similar to the larger sample of clients referred to substance abuse services (Table 2.1), although more women called for an interview, perhaps reflecting women's greater willingness to talk to others about their illness.

The sample is not random, and hence cannot be used to generalize beyond the population of subjects enrolled in the SAMHSA integration project. However, the data is useful in obtaining insights into the many challenges faced by HIV-positive individuals with substance abuse problems. The data is organized by the key themes that emerged from responses to the questions posed by the Kleinman Illness Narratives (Appendix A). The main purpose of the interview is to understand how individuals think about their illness, which is important to understanding barriers to care and treatment.

The first question in the Kleinman Illness Narratives asks clients, "How do you refer to your illness when you talk about it, or think about it?" I expected a great deal of denial or avoidance, and this was evident in a number of responses.[1]

WF66.   "Well, to be honest, I don't refer to it at all—At one time I was in denial; now I pray about it."
RJ65.   "I don't think about it. Go about my everyday life."
AC68.   "I don't call it nothing; I never gave it a name."
BD64.   "It is what it is."
PM59.   "I didn't accept it, now my family knows."
CH68.   "Um . . . I really don't know . . ."
WF66.   "Nothing . . . Life."
AL63.   "Not good."

Obviously, denial of one's HIV status is a major barrier to treatment. However, 12 of the 43 individuals interviewed referred to their illness as HIV, or HIV-positive, or "I've got the virus," or AIDS (one). Another respondent referred to HIV as "my disease . . . I don't really like to say the word." One eloquent man referred to his illness as HIV, but would not use the term in talking to others: "I make up any excuse to keep from telling people that I'm dying from HIV." These responses are also indicative of an

Table 2.1 Summary of Client Demographic Data (Percentages)

	Intake N = 320	6 Month N = 229	12 Month N = 176	Personal Interview N = 43
Gender				
Male	60.3	58.1	56.8	50.0
Female	38.4	41.0	42.6	50.0
Transgender	.6	.9	.6	na
Race				
Black	82.8	82.5	83.5	88.0
White	15.9	15.7	14.8	12.0
Hispanic	.6	.4	.6	–
Am. Indian	.6	.4	.1	–
Housing				
Own Place	41.9	37.7	46.9	
Family/Friends	38.4	37.7	37.7	
Shelter	3.4	3.5	2.9	
Street	3.8	1.3	2.9	
Institution	6.9	3.9	1.7	
½ way house	1.6	6.1	5.1	
Res. Trt	1.9	3.5	1.7	
Other	2.2	1.3	1.1	
Education				
LT High School	46.9	47.6	48.9	
High School	31.3	30.1	25.6	
GT High School	21.8	22.2	25.6	
Employment				
No	22.8	19.2	20.6	
Yes	7.5	14.8	17.1	
Seeking Work	10.6	8.7	6.9	
Disabled	59.1	57.2	55.4	
Health				
Poor	35.0	18.9	17.2	
Fair	33.9	33.3	25.3	
Good	26.9	29.8	33.3	
Very Good	10.8	14.5	15.5	
Excellent	3.5	3.5	8.6	

acceptance of HIV as a medical condition, and another six respondents also referred to their HIV disease as a "sickness" or "condition." Close to half of the respondents had a medical view of HIV as an illness, which is likely to positively affect their acceptance of HIV medications and other treatment recommendations.

What was most interesting, and important in terms of the mental health consequences of HIV disease, is that the other half of the respondents responded by describing how they felt about their HIV illness. Several said they felt "hurt" or "disappointed" and four more respondents specifically said they felt "sad" and "depressed." A couple individuals could not put their feelings into words, exemplified by the following quotes:

MH61: "If there was such a word for another emotion, I'd be looking for it."
WT60: "An experience, emotional, physical, spiritual."
TB63: "Well, it's kind of . . . makes me feel . . . caught in the mix. Given something you didn't deserve; I think about it all the time."

The second question in the Kleinman Illness Narratives asks respondents to describe what "you think your illness does." Reponses to this question also demonstrate a fairly coherent understanding of HIV disease as a physical illness that affects the immune system, or the respondents overall health and physical status, or that they needed to take medications. In describing the severity of their illness, many respondents once again used medical language, saying that their blood levels or CD4 counts were low, or that it's "not bad, I'm not on meds yet" (EL60) or "I'm to the point where I have to take meds every day for the rest of my life" (TM60).

Several respondents directly referred to the experience of their illness with the phrase made famous by Kathy Charmaz (1991), referring to good days and bad days.

WL71: "Um . . . it's different every day; good days, bad days."
RG68: "Some days good; some bad."
AC68: "Sometimes I'm in a good mood; sometimes I'm not."

In describing the severity of their illness, while many referred directly to blood levels or CD4 counts, most simply said either "it's bad" or "it's not too bad." JH56 described the severity of his illness as "Not the best, but not bad." Once again, a number used emotional descriptors to describe their illness: it "causes me to be scared" (JM60); it "takes a lot out of my life" (YB57); it "brings tears to my eyes" (WT61); it "sometimes makes you lonely, it isolates you" (TM60).

When asked about what kind of treatment respondents thought they should receive, many mentioned problems with depression. "I have lots of problems with depression, it's not an illness, but it's a contributing factor . . . I need more psych work" (BS69). Four other individuals targeted a lack of mental health care providers as a problem in their treatment. In a later open-ended question, I asked respondents if they would see a mental health provider if they could, and everyone responded yes.

Throughout the Kleinman Interview Narratives, respondents mentioned loneliness, isolation, and a lack of companionship as problems they experienced because of the illness. Other researchers have also examined the role of what they refer to as "chronic sorrow" (Lichtenstein, Laska, & Clair, 2002), highlighting the importance of social supports. Respondents were then asked "Do you have anyone you can talk to about your problems with your illness or medications?" Close to half indicated they did have someone they could talk to, most often family. PM59 not only "has a supportive family. I talk to my nieces to educate them; to protect themselves." Some individuals had family, but they weren't really supportive: "My family— they're cool; but they don't like talking about it; my ex is the same" (WL71). Nine of the 43 respondents admitted they had no one to talk to; either not responding (3) or responding "no" or "nobody personally." The majority (16) referred to a health care provider, most often their case manager, social worker, or a doctor, as the one they could talk to about their illness. As nicely summarized by MH61, "Hmmm . . . my doctor. So many people still don't understand what's going on. They're in a world of their own. It's the stigma." In a follow up question, almost everyone felt they could talk to their health care providers about their problems, and several referred to their health care providers as "family." Case managers were most often cited as those who meet clients' needs and helped them out most, and I will talk about the role of case managers in the following chapter. The qualitative data gives us insight into the emotional problems faced by individuals living with HIV, as well as the need for social supports, I turn next to a quantitative assessment of mental health and substance use issues, and the role of social supports among the larger group of HIV-positive individuals referred for substance abuse services.

HIV DISEASE AND CO-OCCURRING SUBSTANCE ABUSE AND MENTAL HEALTH PROBLEMS

Who are the individuals living with HIV and receiving care? Data collected from clients referred for enhanced substance abuse services provide one snapshot. I focus on the intake data collected from 320 clients (Table 2.1). The majority are male (60%), and over 80% are African American (for comparison, in 2009, 75% of new HIV cases in Mecklenburg County were male and over 70% of new HIV infections in Mecklenburg County were among African Americans). The majority are stably housed, with close to 42% living in their own place, and another 38% living with either family or friends. Relatively few were homeless or lived in a shelter (7.2%), and 10.2% lived in some sort of institution or treatment facility. Almost half lack a high school diploma, and close to 60% are disabled. They are poor, with the overwhelming majority lacking significant income. The average monthly income including all sources (earned income, disability, family and friends) was only $441.68 (range of 0 to $2,140). Physical health status was also fairly poor, with close to 70% reporting their health was either poor or just fair.

Not surprising, given the fact that HIV-positive clients had been referred for substance abuse treatment, close to 70% (n = 218) had used alcohol or illegal drugs in the past 30 days (Table 2.2), and only seven of these admitted to injecting drugs. However, use of alcohol or drugs was not that typically associated with someone with a substance abuse problem; the mean number of days each month using a substance was only 16.5 (with a standard error of .96), and substance use reduced to just under 9 days at the 6-month follow up, and to just under 7 days a month at the 12-month follow up. While many reported stress or emotional problems due to their substance use, close to half did not feel their substance abuse limited their usual activities (Table 2.3). In sum, patterns of substance use among respondents do not seem to warrant enhanced substance abuse treatment, but concerns over the physical impacts of HIV disease and the need for strict adherence to medications justify efforts to limit even normative patterns of substance use.

In terms of mental health problems, in the past 30 days, 71.8% of the respondents reported they had experienced serious depression, another 61.4% serious anxiety, and 42.9% had trouble thinking or concentrating. Hallucinations or difficulty controlling violent behavior was reported by 11.6 and 12.9% of the respondents, and relatively few had attempted suicide (5.3%). Close to one third had been prescribed psychiatric medication in the past 30 days. As with substance use, respondents reported improvements to their mental health over the course of the study: The mean number of days experiencing depression, anxiety, and or trouble concentrating and thinking dropped from 34.7 days at intake, to 27.75 days at the 6-month follow up, to 18.3 days at the 12-month follow up.

Table 2.3 provides information on adherence and social supports, supplemental questions that were added to the SAMHSA data collection instrument. Unfortunately, staff collecting data dropped these questions in year three (a new coordinator was hired who decided to make the questionnaire shorter by eliminating all questions not required by SAMHSA). Consequently, the number of respondents is smaller (n = 154), although the data still allow us to track changes over time. We had ascertained in an earlier adherence study (see Chapter 5) that the primary reasons to stop taking medications for chronic conditions is either the medications make individuals feel sick or have unpleasant side effects, or the individuals start to feel better and no longer feel they need the medications. At intake, close to half of respondents (46.7%) admitted they stopped taking their HIV medications because they made them feel worse, while 35.5% stopped

Table 2.2 Behavioral Data at Intake, 6 month and 12 month (Percentages)

	Intake (n = 320)	6 Month (N = 229)	12 Month (n = 176)
Used Alcohol or Illegal Drugs in past 30 days			
No	31.9	56.3	65.3
Yes	68.1	53.7	34.7
Stress Due to Substance Use			
Not at all	31.8	50.0	59.7
Somewhat	19.6	21.4	18.8
Considerable	11.9	9.7	5.8
Extremely	36.7	18.9	15.6
Extent Substance Abuse Caused Limitations to Usual Activities			
Not at all	47.6	64.8	73.4
Somewhat	16.1	14.3	11.0
Considerable	10.3	5.6	4.5
Extremely	26.0	15.3	11.0
Extent Bothered by Emotional Problems Due to Substance Use			
Not at all	38.3	56.6	69.0
Somewhat	20.6	19.9	14.8
Considerable	13.8	6.1	3.9
Extremely	27.3	17.3	12.3
Experienced Emotional Problems Not Due to Substance Use (in past 30 days)			
Serious Depression	71.8	56.8	48.3
Serious Anxiety	61.4	52.0	44.3
Trouble Thinking	42.9	32.6	23.6
Hallucinations	11.6	6.5	5.2
Control Violent Beh.	12.9	9.3	6.3
Attempted Suicide	5.3	1.3	.6
Prescribed Meds	29.8	26.4	19.0

Mean Number of Days (s.d) in past 30 days R experienced serious depression, serious anxiety, and/or had trouble thinking, concentrating, or remembering.

	34.66 (2.0)	27.75 (2.2)	18.26 (1.9)

taking their HIV medications because they were feeling better. However, adherence improved considerably over the course of the study. Levels of social support were fairly high: 60% had a main partner, and this person helped almost 80% of these individuals cope. Most felt close to family and/or

Table 2.3 Adherence and Social Support (Note: N's are smaller, as these were supplemental questions that were not asked during year 3)

	Intake N = 254	6 Month N = 198	12 Month N = 137
Cut back or stopped taking HIV meds because they made you feel worse			
No	53.4	73.7	72.5
Yes	46.7	26.3	24.8
Stopped taking HIV meds as you were feeling better			
No	64.5	76.3	79.4
Yes	35.5	23.7	20.6
Main Partner			
No	61.8	62.1	56.3
Yes	38.2	37.9	43.7
Partner Helps You Cope			
No	21.8	15.8	22.1
Yes (a little to a lot)	78.2	84.2	77.9
Feels Close to Family/Friends			
No	17.5	14.6	9.6
Sometimes	19.1	13.6	8.1
Yes	63.3	71.7	82.2
Gets Practical Help from Family/Friends			
No	17.5	16.7	10.3
Sometimes	13.9	8.6	6.6
Yes	68.7	74.7	83.1
Can Talk to Family/Friends			
No	21.8	13.1	14.7
Sometimes	15.1	13.6	8.8
Yes	63.1	73.2	76.5
Family/Friends Know My HIV Status			
No	13.9	10.7	11.8
Some Do	11.5	9.1	2.9
Yes	74.6	80.2	85.3
Family/Friends have Substance Abuse Problems			
No	25.8	25.8	20.6
Some Do	7.9	7.1	5.1
Yes	66.3	67.2	74.3

friends (63.3%), received practical help from family/friends (68.7%), could talk to family/friends (63.1%), and the majority of family/friends were aware of the HIV status of the client (74.6%). However, individuals in these social support networks also had substance abuse problems (66.3%), a factor in respondents' own continued use of substances despite being HIV-positive.

In terms of demographic differences in substance abuse and mental health problems (Table 2.4), there were no differences between men and women regarding substance abuse, but women were more likely to experience mental health problems at intake. African Americans were more likely to report substance use, while Whites had more mental health problems. In Table 2.5, I examine the predictors of mental health problems at intake. Race and gender differences are not significant predictors; instead, social support (an additive scale of having a partner and support from family/friends) is critical, with those having more social support reporting fewer mental health problems. Adherence is also significant—individuals who were non-adherent to their HIV medications were more likely to experience mental health problems. Poor physical health was also associated with more days with mental health problems.

Table 2.6 provides a causal analysis of the experience of mental health problems (operationalized in days as described above) and substance use (once again, in days) at the 6-month follow up (controlling for mental health problems and substance use at intake), and Table 2.7 provides the same analysis for the 12-month follow up. As one would expect, previous mental

Table 2.4 Demographic Differences in Mental Health and Substance Abuse Problems (means, S.D)

	Male	Female	White	Black
Mental Health Problems:				
Intake	31.3 (29.3)	39.8 (44.5)	38.1 (29.2)	33.8 (37.4)
	p = .040		p = .446	
6 Month	24.7 (28.7)	31.8 (39.8)	29.5 (30.9)	27.2 (34.4)
	p = .122		p = .712	
12 Month	18.4 (24.5)	18.4 (26.6)	30.1 (33.4)	15.9 (23.0)
	p = .997		p = .008	
Substance Use:				
Intake	17.2 (17.6)	15.0 (16.5)	9.9 (12.1)	17.7 (17.9)
	p = .274		p = .004	
6 Month	9.7 (16.3)	8.1 (12.6)	7.9 (14.5)	9.2 (15.0)
	p = .412		p = .630	
12 Month	7.9 (13.3)	5.9 (11.2)	8.7 (17.2)	6.5 (11.5)
	p = .311		p = .400	

Table 2.5 Multivariate Analysis of Mental Health Problems at Intake (n = 241)

Variables	B	Std. Error	Beta	p-value
Race (1 = Black)	−4.99	5.88	−.053	.396
Gender (1 = female)	3.20	4.34	.047	.461
Years Education	−.927	1.01	−.058	.362
Health (5 = excellent)	−3.35	2.03	−.107	.100
Social Support (0-7)	−2.02	.939	−.137	.032
Non Adherence (1 = yes)	10.134	4.30	.150	.019
R-Square		.076	.005	

Table 2.6 Multivariate Analysis of Behavioral Outcomes at 6 Months (n = 223)

Variables	Mental Health Problem			Substance Use		
	B	SE	p-value	B	SE	p-value
Race	−.028	5.79	.658	.002	2.70	.980
Gender	.001	4.48	.990	−.082	2.09	.238
Education	−.106	1.01	.099	−.058	.475	.397
Health, 6 m	−.266	2.00	.000	−.196	.938	.004
Days MH, intake	.277	.056	.000	−.006	.026	.932
Days SA, intake	−.048	.130	.452	.113	.061	.051
R-Square	.173		.000	.163		.001

Table 2.7 Multivariate Analysis of Behavioral Outcomes at 12 Months (n = 145)

Variables	Mental Health Problem			Substance Use		
	B	SE	p-value	B	SE	p-value
Race	−.223	5.54	.004	−.078	2.83	.330
Gender	−.039	4.107	.625	−.028	2.10	.740
Education	.071	.967	.376	−.039	.495	.641
Health, 12 m	−.397	1.81	.000	−.135	.926	.101
Days MH, 6 m	.185	.056	.020	−.071	.029	.389
Days SA, 6 m	−.104	.155	.183	.355	.079	.000
Visits, SA	.033	.148	.670	−.069	.076	.392
R-Square	.234		.000	.163		.001

health problems predicted mental health problems at each follow up, and previous substance use predicted subsequent substance use. However, physical health status (measured at the time of the follow up) was the only factor found to predict both mental health problems and substance use—poor physical health led to both more days with mental health problems and more substance use.

While social support was not a significant predictor at the 6- or 12-month follow up, it was at intake. Social support can also improve adherence, and ultimately physical health, improving mental health and reducing substance use. Social support can also enhance self-esteem, and help combat the isolating effects of stigma.

PEER BASED SOCIAL SUPPORTS

Peer based social support programs have the potential to serve as ongoing sources of social support for individuals living with HIV disease, as they can augment more traditional social supports, and can also serve as an important avenue to increase advocacy and empowerment. Peer support is not therapy; rather, peers help individuals living with HIV meet practical problems of living, share knowledge, and are available when needed. Peer support programs work by providing necessary social support, either helping consumers meet basic needs (instrumental support), socio-emotional support (providing a sense of belonging or friendship), or enhancing recreational skills and thus promoting community integration. Peer support enhances self-management and problem solving strategies, and can lead to higher levels of empowerment (Clay, Schell, Corrigan, & Ralph, 2005). Cunningham, Sanchez, Li, Heller, and Sohler (2008) found that social support groups lead to higher utilization of HIV health related services. In-depth interviews with 20 patients who had sustained undetectable viral loads revealed that these consumers found a lack of social support to be the greatest hindrance for them, and fostering beneficial relationships to be most helpful (Alfonso, Geller, Bermbach, Drummond, & Montaner, 2006). Peer support provides for helpful relationships and thereby enhances social support.

There is substantial literature on peer support programs for those living with mental illness (Clay et al., 2005; Neugeboren, 1999), and literature on both the challenges and benefits of peer based interventions for individuals living with HIV disease (Raja et al., 2008). Peer interventions have been successful in HIV prevention and outreach (Broadhead et al., 2002; Latkin et al., 2009) and peer support has been found to improve quality of life (Molassiotis, Callaghan, Twinn, Lam, & Chung, 2002) and hope (Harris & Larson, 2007). There is literature that explores how best to provide peer support and how to tailor peer support for diversity (Hilfinger, Moneyham, Vyavaharkar, Murdaugh, & Phillips, 2009; Messias, Moneyham, Murdaugh, & Phillips, 2006).

HIV service providers can help facilitate the development of peer based social supports for their clients. There is consensus that comprehensive HIV care requires integrated interventions (Stoff, Mitnick, & Kalichman, 2004) and multidisciplinary collaboration (Soto, Bell, & Pillen, 2004). In addition, consumers and providers need to be active partners in treatment (Stoff et al., 2004). This HIV Cost Study (HIV/AIDS Treatment Adherence, Health Outcomes and Cost Study Group, 2004) used multidisciplinary treatment teams and consumer advisory groups to deliver care to multiply diagnosed individuals living with HIV disease. These groups can empower clients and train them to work within the system to provide support and services to other clients.

However, recent funding restrictions have reduced the opportunities for social support groups and peer based interventions. In Mecklenburg County, key agencies that offered social support groups directed to specialized populations have ceased to exist. Changes in Ryan White funding have also limited the social support role of HIV case managers. In response to the closing of one of the major HIV provider agencies, which provided case management to over 600 clients, and numerous social support groups, the Mecklenburg HIV Council conducted a community forum in January 2008. I return to the voices of clients, who spoke eloquently at this forum about their need for social supports and how the closing of this particular agency would affect their lives. One long-term survivor of the system (as she referred to herself) spoke movingly:

> I wanted someone to take it away, to wake up from this nightmare. I was a porcelain doll; I was shattered. I suffered a 3-year depression. I needed someone with superglue to put me together; I need a safe place, a family where I am accepted and loved. (Name of Agency) did that.

Another consumer also referred to this agency as her "only family. They helped me understand why I need meds; I learned a lot from other people in my group."

A much younger Black woman who had lived with HIV for 12 years described her need for social supports:

> I need a lot of support. I need to hear that you are there for me. There are days when I'm tired, when I stumble. I need some encouragement. I need to be more than a number. I need individual attention. I don't want to die alone.

Providers attending the forum were also frustrated. While the increased Ryan White funding for medical services was "great, that's not all of it. It's more than seeing the doctor. It's more than medications. People's basic needs have to be met." Another provider (a nurse) emphasized the importance of case management in enhancing clients' mental health by providing for ongoing support, and that this kind of social support is critical to survival and treatment success.

In response to limited funding for ongoing social supports, local service agencies have sponsored a number of peer support and advocacy work-shops, and have sought funding for peer support programs and multidisci-plinary treatment teams, which were not ultimately funded. The Regional HIV/AIDS Consortium did partner with Duke University and obtained a 2-year exploratory grant that provides in-house mental health counseling for 40 clients. Furthermore, consumers who have made the transition from client to provider have played an instrumental role in developing alternative social support groups. One such client turned provider described her role, "It's been a growing experience. It is therapeutic that I can help put oth-ers back together. I have the glue in my hands." These consumer/providers have become more public in their criticism of gaps in the service system. One social support group, Positive Connections, was formed in response to Ryan White requirements for a consumer advisory council. This group has also become increasingly vocal, and elicited the support of key elected officials. Providers have also recognized that they need to teach their clients to advocate for themselves. Kielmann and Cataldo (2011) describe the role of such "expert" patients, as allowing for greater self-management, as well as advocacy. In the next chapter, I turn to the work of case managers, who so often are the clients' only "family," and whose work involves advocacy on behalf of their clients.

NOTE

1. ID represents initials and year of birth.

3 Advocating for My Client
Treatment Ideologies and Barriers to Integrated Care

INTRODUCTION

In this chapter, I examine the work of HIV case managers. While individuals living with HIV have a doctor—often an infectious disease doctor—their primary source of professional support often comes from their case manager. Case management is the most fundamental means of integrating care at the client level. A case manager coordinates the various services and supports needed by the client, and also provides both emotional and tangible social supports (Dill, 2001). With clients who are HIV-positive, case managers must also educate the clients about their treatment and medications, advocate for their clients, and help them overcome barriers to care (Ross-Friend, Schuster, & Sherry, 2011). Cunningham, Wong, and Hays (2008) found that having a case manager significantly improved physical health for a nationally representative sample of HIV-positive clients receiving care in the HIV Costs and Services Utilization Study.

The majority of the individuals interviewed in Chapter 2 identified their case managers as the health providers they had the closest relationship with. Case management can be performed by anyone with some professional preparation or background in human services work. While case management is generally not deemed as professionally challenging or rewarding as more clearly defined clinical work (such as nursing, social work, or counseling), it does involve a high degree of emotional involvement and a diverse skill set, especially given the multiple needs of clients who are HIV-positive. Case managers must ensure their clients receive medically necessary services; keep track of their clients' CD4 counts, viral loads, and adherence to complicated medication regimes; ensure clients' basic needs (housing, income supports, etc.) are being met; and provide for social supports. In addition, case managers need to be aware of and try to deal proactively with the substance use and mental health problems of their clients. Case managers report that the support they provide can improve their clients' quality of life (Chernesky & Grube, 1999), and clients whose case managers helped them cope with depression have been found to have higher quality of life (Pugh, 2009).

I begin this chapter by first providing a demographic profile of a typical health care provider serving clients with identified HIV risk, mental health, and substance abuse problems, utilizing data I collected in 2001 as part of a needs assessment. I then turn to a more in-depth examination of the work of HIV case managers. The Ryan White CARE Act of 1990 included funding for case management services, and oversight over case management activities often fell to the HIV/AIDS Consortium authorized by Ryan White dollars. Such has been the case in Charlotte. With the reauthorization of the Ryan White CARE Act, case management has been strictly defined to focus only on the provision of medically necessary services—this is a point I will return to later. In fulfilling its role, the Regional HIV/AIDS Consortium in Charlotte had a case manager coordinator who provided training of case managers, conducted checks on the files and charts kept by HIV case managers, held regular meetings with case managers, and provided general oversight to the activities of case managers who operated in a number of different agencies in the 13-county area overseen by the Regional HIV/AIDS Consortium.

BACKGROUND AND COMPETENCIES OF HEALTH CARE PROVIDERS

In September 2001, I conducted a survey of health care providers in order to determine what kinds of skills and training they needed to provide comprehensive HIV care (this was done in order to justify support for the cross-trainings described in Chapter 5; no funding was provided for the research). A questionnaire was distributed to 75 direct care providers using the mailing list from the local Area Health Education Center (AHEC). The list contained over 1,200 names, and a simple random sample was drawn. The mailing list included providers serving clients at risk for HIV/AIDS with mental health and/or substance abuse problems. The 24 providers who responded (a 32% response rate) had all received additional training in HIV/AIDS, mental health, substance abuse, or cultural competency, and 52.2% had participated in previous cross-trainings offered by AHEC. The majority of these providers (60.9%) had been in their current positions over 5 years, and most said they would also stay in their current positions if they were free to choose (50.9%). Consequently, the questionnaire was completed by providers familiar with the needs of clients with HIV/AIDS, MH, and SA problems.

Respondents were representative of the population of providers in the AHEC mailing list. The majority were female (78%), 65% were White, 30% were African American, and 4.3% were Hispanic. The majority (73.9%) were in the non-profit sector. Providers reported that close to half of their clients are at risk for HIV/AIDS (although only 7.5% were known to be HIV-positive), 41% had a substance abuse problem, 51% had mental health problems, and 41% were estimated to be at risk for all three health problems. Of the respondents' clients, 39% were White, 51% African American, 7% Hispanic, and less than 1% Asian or American Indian (close to 1% were other ethnic groups). However, only 6.4% of these clients had difficulty speaking English. Close to 16% of the providers had some proficiency in Spanish, but the majority (73.7%) were not able to converse in any other language besides English.

In terms of providers' ability to provide care to these clients, the majority (78.3%) reported being able to see a new client referred to them within a week. The major sources of delay would be in not being able to get in touch with the client, a lack of time, or having a full caseload. The majority (61%) had assessment tools for more than one health care problem (HIV/AIDS, MH, or SA) while 21.7% reported no assessment tools for HIV/AIDS, MH, or SA. An equal number of providers (8.7%) had tools to assess mental health or substance abuse. The majority (69.6%) reported that their clients were sometimes or often in need of treatment **not** covered by their insurance. The biggest barriers faced by their clients were a lack of access to resources for daily living (47.4%), lack of health care resources (31.6%), lack of family or social support (10.5%), and problems with multicultural or immigrant status (10.5%).

Responses to the questions to assess service system coordination are presented in Table 3.1; these questions were drawn from the SAMSHA Treatment Improvement Protocol Series, Number 37 (Center for Substance Abuse Treatment (CSAT), 2000). Responses were in the middle range of a scale from "never" to "always," indicating that respondents were somewhat aware of agencies that could meet the various needs of clients, and they felt there were culturally appropriate support groups for clients. Respondents were less familiar with physicians and clinics that accepted HIV-positive clients, with agencies that administer Ryan White funds or how these funds could be used, with eligibility guides for the State's AIDS drug assistance program, or with other forms of financial support that might be available to clients. When averaging the responses to system integration, providers who had attended cross-training sessions reported higher scores (2.43 with an s.d. of .468) than providers who had not attended cross-training sessions (2.12 with an s.d. of .66).

Questions to assess multicultural competence were taken from the October 1999 report, *Overcoming Barriers to Providing Culturally Competent Healthcare*, from the Healthcare Task Force of the Mayor's International Cabinet in Charlotte, North Carolina, and are also reported in Table 3.2. Once again, responses are in the middle range, although the means are lower and the percentage of respondents selecting "Never" is much higher, indicating that multicultural competence is lower overall than system integration. It is evident there is an organizational commitment to multiculturalism, and an awareness of the importance of cultural competence and accessibility. However, direction and information signs were generally not available, nor were consent forms, discharge instructions, satisfaction surveys, or other

Table 3.1 Service System Integration. Responses ranged from 0 (never) to 4 (always). Means and Standard Deviations are reported. Percentages responding NEVER are also included.

	Mean (S.D)	% NEVER
1. I am familiar with those area physicians and clinics with experience in HIV/AIDS issues and who accept HIV-positive patients.	1.74 (.81)	0%
2. I know what HIV/AIDS service organizations exist in this community.	2.87 (.81)	0%
3. I know who administers Ryan White funds, and how these funds can be used.	1.04 (1.36)	47.8%
4. I know where an individual with HIV/AIDS can obtain mental health services.	2.91 (1.08)	0%
5. I know where an individual with HIV/AIDS can obtain substance abuse services.	3.35 (.98)	0%
6. I know how to obtain medical coverage for patients who are indigent or for undocumented workers.	2.30 (1.26)	8.7%
7. Area substance abuse treatment programs are prepared to deal with a client's complicated HIV/AIDS treatment regiment.	2.32 (.82)	0%
8. There are mental health programs which can provide psychiatric evaluation, medication management, or case management for clients with mental health problems.	3.14 (.99)	0%
9. I am familiar with the eligibility guidelines for the state's AIDS Drug Assistance Program, and know which drugs are covered by the program.	1.09 (1.11)	31.8%
10. There are culturally appropriate local support groups available for persons living with HIV/AIDS.	2.71 (1.01)	4.8%
11. There are culturally appropriate local support groups available for persons living with substance abuse disorders.	2.32 (.99)	4.5%
12. There are culturally appropriate local support groups available for persons living with mental illness.	2.32 (1.13)	9.1%
13. I know what forms of financial assistance are available to clients to pay for HIV/AIDS treatment.	1.55 (1.18)	18.2%
14. I know what forms of support are available to help with loss, death, and dying.	2.73 (1.03)	4.5%
15. I am able to link my clients to needed housing and social supports in the community.	2.45 (1.14)	9.1%

Table 3.2 Cultural Competency. Responses ranged from 0 (never) to 4 (always). Means and Standard Deviations are reported. Percentages responding NEVER are also included.

	Mean (S.D)	%
1. There are written policies in place which address the needs of the non-English speaking populations in this community.	2.57 (1.25)	9.5%
2. Policies, procedures, and guidelines are currently in place to evaluate the need for an interpreter.	2.67 (1.24)	9.5%
3. When a patient who does not speak English pre-schedules an appointment, we make special provisions ahead of time for an interpreter.	3.09 (1.57)	18.2%
4. Directions and information signs displayed incorporate the major languages spoken in our community.	1.59 (1.37)	27.3%
5. Children or minors are not used to interpret or translate medical client information.	1.09 (1.44)	54.5%
6. Informed consent including treatment, diagnostic, financial information, research and Patients' Rights documents are available in all major languages.	1.81 (1.25)	28.6%
7. Discharge instructions and information regarding medical appointments are written simply in the major languages spoken in our community.	2.00 (1.59)	30.0%
8. Staff training and education has been presented on cultural diversity issues, such as the prevailing beliefs, customs, and values of the ethnic communities we serve.	2.32 (1.09)	4.5%
9. There are materials and resources in major languages and an agency glossary of technical and healthcare terms that can be used for interpreting and translations.	1.50 (1.22)	27.3%
10. Written policies and procedures are in place to protect the confidentiality of the non-English speaking client.	2.38 (1.40)	14.3%
11. Client satisfaction surveys and grievance procedures are available in all major languages.	1.52 (1.25)	28.6%
12. Non-English speaking clients are informed on how to communicate their concerns to a representative in our organization.	1.77 (1.19)	18.2%
13. Information and community resources on interpreter services are up to date, on site, and accessible to employees.	2.55 (1.24)	13.6%
14. The reception areas in our healthcare setting includes magazines and books that reflect the ethnic communities we currently serve.	1.73 (1.42)	27.3%

(Continued)

Table 3.2 (Continued)

	Mean (S.D)	%
15. When a client enters our system for services, there is an admission database which includes an assessment of a client's cultural identity and healthcare practices.	2.27 (1.39)	18.2%
16. There is a process in place to assess the ability of non-English speaking clients to read and understand documents that are written in their native language.	1.55 (1.32)	30.0%
17. Family members and friends are rarely used as interpreters in our healthcare setting.	1.14 (1.11)	33.3%
18. Bilingual members of our staff have been given training on medical terminology and can serve as interpreters.	1.05 (1.63)	28.6%
19. Our organization is actively recruiting multilingual, multi-cultural healthcare professionals.	2.50 (1.47)	13.6%
20. There is a process in place to assess the competency of interpreters and translators.	2.19 (1.54)	19.0%

materials and resources available in languages other than English. Reception areas did not include reading materials in languages other than English, nor were there processes in place to assess the English speaking ability of clients. Furthermore, bilingual staff members were generally not given training on medical terminology so they could serve as translators.

This data, drawn from all types of health providers, provides a frame for understanding the work of HIV case managers. With funding from SAMHSA for the Enhanced Substance Abuse Project (described in Chapter 2), quarterly meetings were held with HIV case managers and substance abuse providers. I collected data from these providers at each spring meeting beginning in 2003 and ending in 2007 (the years of the SAMHSA funding). While required of HIV case managers, there are relatively few individuals who completed the survey in multiple years; the high turnover of case managers is apparent with the relative low numbers of individuals who were repeats, especially in 2006 and 2007. In 2003, 22 individuals completed the questionnaire and six of these also completed the questionnaire in subsequent years. Table 3.3 provides a summary of the number completing the survey each year, as well as "repeats," and provides information on the professional background of case managers.[1] Case managers were primarily women, African American, and while most had a college degree, the proportion with an advanced degree (either MSW, RN, or other Master's level degree) was relatively small.

The questionnaire contained fixed-choice questions about respondents' training and training needs, knowledge of the system, cultural competence, psychological burnout, and work satisfaction. In addition, open-ended

Table 3.3   Case Manager Cross-Training, Respondents by Year

Year of Survey	2003	2004	2005	2006	2007
N	22	25	10	25	16
N Repeats	–	2	4	4	2
MA	4	4	2	3	1
MSW	1	1	0	0	2
Nursing[a]	5	7	3	4	1
BA	9	10	4	14	11
Work Exper.[b]	3	0	1	4	1

[a] Includes all individuals with any nursing degree; however, only 3 individuals over the 5 years were RNs, with one of these individuals participating in 4 cross-trainings.

[b] Individuals did not specify a degree, only relevant work experience, so one can assume they did not have a college degree but had met job qualifications based upon their years of work experience in the field.

questions asked for more detailed information about their work, relationships with clients, barriers to performing their work, and suggestions as to how the system could be improved. I rely on the open-ended questions in this chapter to examine (a) providers' work with HIV clients, (b) their treatment ideologies, and (c) barriers to care.

ADVOCATING FOR HIV CLIENTS

HIV case managers (referred to hereafter simply as providers) often described their role as that of being an advocate for their clients, and this is a key ingredient to the definition of case management most often assessed by HIV case managers (CSAT, 1998). Many providers included the descriptor of friend in their elaboration of the advocacy role. The centrality of the advocacy role comes out clearly when I asked providers to describe a critical incident (Benner, 1984). The question was worded as follows:

> Think about an incident, or story, that sticks out in your mind about your work.
>   This story or incident could be one in which your intervention made a difference, an incident that went unusually well, or an incident where things did not go as planned. Describe the incident (please do not include any identifying information in your response to this question). Why was the incident critical? What were your concerns?

This question was only asked in 2006 and 2007, and since 2007 contained the most detailed responses from the individuals who completed the questionnaire, I will use that year to describe providers' advocacy role and their relationships with their clients. Of the 16 providers who completed the questionnaire, 10 answered the critical incident question (perhaps as part of their aversion to paperwork, case managers were often reluctant to complete open-ended questions).

To begin, only two of the critical incidents described a positive story. When I collected the same type of data from mental health providers in the 1990s, the critical incidents were fairly evenly split between negative and positive stories (Scheid, 2004b). Given the many needs of HIV clients and the high levels of poverty and lack of support (Chapter 2), it is not surprising that critical incidents are overwhelmingly negative. But let us begin with a truly remarkable story—where a young HIV-positive woman becomes an advocate herself, one of those "expert patients" identified by Kielmann and Cataldo (2010):

> I had a 23-year-old White female who found out she was HIV positive after giving birth to her daughter who is also HIV positive. At first, she was dumbfounded and in denial, as well as depressed due to the fact that had it passed on to her baby. When we did the DNA testing through the prenatal fluid, it was her ex-boyfriend who had given her HIV, as well as impregnated her. He was notified, tested, and too was in denial. After speaking to this young woman and discussing all of the variables, she agreed and consented to mental health treatment and attended support groups. She also gave consent for her daughter for treatment, as well. Today, she is in college, very compliant, has her own transportation and apartment. Her daughter is doing well, too! The best part of this is that she is an advocate for young HIV-positive women and a speaker.
>
> (BA trained community health worker, LL)

This story provides insight into the diversity of roles a good case manager must assume. First there is medical intervention, then establishing a relationship and linking the client to other forms of social support (in this case, mental health, as well as social support groups), and then helping the client move on to a more autonomous existence (housing, transportation, education).

The negative stories reflect clients in pain, facing almost insurmountable obstacles. In some cases, the case manager is able to do something; in others, there is little the case manager can do. The following critical incident shows how hard providers must advocate for their clients in order for them to obtain even the most basic supports.

> One client was diagnosed with HIV/AIDS in August '06: no job, no insurance, no money. He lives with his wonderful mother who works and supports her son. I have helped him to navigate the SSD system and the Medicaid system. I have also helped him with patient assistance programs. He was denied disability and Medicaid. I helped him appeal the Medicaid and the decision was reversed. I am in the process of helping

him with a reconsideration for disability. He was scared and depressed when I first started working with him. He is now feeling better and is adherent with his medications (he has our adherence RN working with him). He has also been supported by an RN in our health department who was helping him with his TB medication. He has Medicaid now and still awaiting the disability, but is much improved!

(BA HIV case manager, SC)

This story also shows the importance of coordinated care; the client has an adherence nurse, as well as another nurse in the health department who helps him with his TB medications. That leaves the case manager free to focus on income supports (a role no longer allowed under the new Ryan White guidelines). However, several other providers show how their provider roles move them into unforeseen types of advocacy. One BSW case manager (CN) had "a client who was admitted into the hospital and, as a result, had her feet amputated. This individual had no insurance and was in the process of losing her housing. I was able to get funding to keep the client's home. I really felt worthwhile after helping her." Another MPH case manager (OO) provided a detailed story about a client who had been accused of smoking crack in the public housing unit where he lived:

My client was informed that they had received a police report stating my client was smoking crack. Client stated that he was given a copy of this "police report." When I saw that the report was actually an email, I became quite infuriated, as it was obvious that officers were taking advantage of the fact that my client was illiterate. I advocated on behalf of my client and because of this, he is still currently in his home.

In both incidents, providers had to advocate for their clients to simply maintain their housing in the face of adversity. Critical incidents from other years of the survey often included descriptions of a case manager finding a client housing.

The negative stories without a happy ending involve either clients who don't qualify for any type of assistance, or who simply do not have any form of social support. For example, JJ, a BSW, reported her "most difficult case is a family with an HIV-positive father that falls squarely in the cracks of all systems. He doesn't qualify for disability, Medicaid, ADAP, patient assistance programs, or housing assistance." An RN nurse (SS) described "a client that has no significant person in his life that will be of any support; I am concerned he may get very ill and there will be no one to look out for his interests."

There is also frustration with clients who are perceived as taking advantage of the systems. This was often listed as a barrier to care, or a common form of stress. While not widely prevalent, the following story of a "con" shows the lengths that case managers will go to in order to meet their clients' needs.

A client and his wife spoke to another case manager for emergency heat assistance; this con ended up with the referral not knowing they spent most of the yearly allotment. They had a power bill cut off notice and this case manager promised it would be paid by EFA funds. They (clients) took forms to other agencies and received no additional funding. As to not go back on a promise, as they had children at home, this case manager ended paying for their entire bill.

(BSW case manager, JR)

We can see from these stories how critical the advocacy role is for HIV case management and to what lengths providers must go to ensure their clients have the most basic forms of support—housing and income. Case managers often referred to Maslow's hierarchy in describing their work with HIV-positive clients—medication compliance and recovery can only come when the more basic needs of housing and income supports are met. I turn next to a more systematic examination of how providers viewed their work, to their treatment ideologies, and concrete goals for their clients.

TREATMENT IDEOLOGIES AND CARE PLANS

Treatment ideology is the complex set of beliefs that health care providers hold about health, illness, and treatment (Scheid, 1994). These beliefs consist of specific theories about the etiology of illness, the role of the patient or client, and the validity or efficacy of various treatments (see Abbott, 1992; Eaton, Ritter, & Brown, 1990; and Strauss, Schatzman, Burcher, Ehrlich, & Sabshin, 1964, for discussions of medical ideologies). Such ideologies guide the treatment decisions and behaviors of providers—they tell the provider what to do and how to do it. Treatment ideologies contain both "is" and "ought" properties, and specify both what a provider can do (operative aspects of ideologies) and what they ought to do under ideal conditions (fundamental aspects of ideologies). Strauss et al. (1964, p. 360) argued that ideologies are mediated by operational philosophies that are "systems of ideas and procedures for implementing therapeutic ideologies under specific institutional conditions." That is, what one would ideally like to do, or feel one ought to do, and what one can realistically do in a given situation may conflict. For example, ideally, treatment for an HIV client would end with the client obtaining medical care, social supports, and becoming an advocate herself (as described in the critical incident above). Realistically, finding and maintaining basic supports such as housing and income or medication adherence may be all the provider can accomplish with existing resources. This conflict between fundamental aspects and operative aspects must be mediated by providers, who need to feel that the care they are providing is effective and that they are doing all they can for the client.

HIV providers come from a wide variety of backgrounds, have different kinds of educational credentials, serve different kinds of clients, and work in different organizations; obviously, their treatment ideologies differ. Yet these providers need to develop common standards of care in order to meet the multiple needs of their triply diagnosed clients. Practical work experiences can shape theoretical belief systems (Benner, 1984) and since HIV providers face may of the same kinds of problems, I would expect to find some consistency in their treatment orientations or ideologies of care. I developed a typology of the treatment ideologies of mental health workers (Scheid, 1994) that is based on two axis, or domain assumptions about two fundamental questions. First, what is the appropriate role for the provider? That is, how is the provider to behave toward the client; how will he/she act? A given role specifies the type of relationship a provider will develop with the client. The second question is: What is the goal of treatment, or what is the intended outcome of treatment? What is the provider working toward? What constitutes success? While there is variability in both treatment role and goal from client to client, in general, providers articulate consistency in their approaches to providing treatment. I found that mental health care providers adhere to treatment ideologies that are consistent with the principles of community-based care: caretaking, re-parenting, normalization, and empowerment (Scheid, 2004b). Treatment ideologies did vary among professional groups, with nurses more likely to adhere to supportive treatment ideologies (caretaking or normalization) and case managers more likely to be facilitative (re-parenting and empowerment).

There were some similarities between the treatment ideologies of HIV providers and mental health providers, but also some important differences. First, in HIV care work, there is much greater emphasis on medication adherence and physical health, as would be expected. Second, HIV case management has not been subject to the same kind of professionalization as mental health and there are no set philosophies of care that are built around causal illness models.[2] I use the data collected in 2004 and 2006 to examine how providers described their role and their treatment goals (there was only one provider who answered these open questions in both years and I simply deleted his 2005 responses from the analysis; as noted above, his responses were almost the same in both years). Combing these years provides an overall sample size of 49, although there are some missing data (five respondents did not identify a role and six did not specify a treatment goal).

There were three overriding roles that captured the diversity of provider responses to the question, "I must assume the role of a _____ (please fill in the blank with a descriptor for how you see your role in the relationship with your clients)." Responses were coded into only one category with no overlap, even though some providers gave multiple descriptors. In these cases, the first descriptor (or the most prevalent of multiple roles) was utilized. Table 3.4 describes the most typical or general roles providers assumed with their clients. In seeking underlying dimensions to

Table 3.4 Descriptive Roles of Case Managers

Role	N	%
Professional Role:		
Counselor or Therapist	9	20.0
Coordinator/coach/educator	7	15.5
Case Manager	6	13.3
Supportive Role:		
Friend/helper	8	17.9
Mother/care giver	5	11.1
Support Person	4	8.9
Advocate	6	13.3
Total	45	100.0

these roles, I identify three predominate role types. First is a provider view of themselves in fairly strict professional terms—that of case manager, counselor, or coordinator/educator. The "professional" constitute the majority of the responses—22 respondents, or 48.9%. Second, providers identified their role as a support person, caregiver, friend, helper, or mother (two respondents included "mother" in their role descriptions). Thirteen respondents (28.9%) identified their primary role as a "supportive" one. Finally, six providers, or 13.3% of the respondents, identified their role as advocates. However, other roles (e.g., compliance and stability) also include advocacy, as described in the critical incidents. It is actually noteworthy that so many described their primary role as advocate.

Next, we turn to the identification of treatment goals. Respondents were asked, "In your opinion, given your existing caseload and client population, what constitutes successful treatment?" This question was worded to arrive at operative (rather than ideal) treatment goals and ideologies. Providers wrote much more in response to this question, yet their responses quickly displayed five different kinds of treatment approaches (Table 3.5) that reflect a continuum of treatment orientations ranging from compliance with medication and treatment, to stability in living situation, to a focus on patient autonomy.[3]

There is a more even distribution of provider ideologies of care in the identification of the treatment goals. A little over a third focused on medication compliance and/or abstinence (with the later being primarily substance abuse providers). Typical responses included "if they are keeping medication appointments and taking meds" or "clients are receiving primary care; have an ID doctor." For a substance abuse provider, successful treatment was "regular meeting attendance, obtaining a sponsor, and long-term sobriety."

Another third of the respondents focused on stability in life situation and getting the client into care, i.e., "getting your client the services they need

Table 3.5   Goals Case Managers Have for HIV Clients

Goal	N	%
Compliance:		
Medication Compliance/Abstinence	14	32.5
Stability:		
Client has needed supports	8	18.6
Client is in care/treatment	7	16.3
Autonomy:		
Good relationship with client/trust	9	20.9
Client is taking care of themselves	5	11.6
Total	43	99.9

in a timely manner," or "engaging them in consistent care," or "stability with housing, employment, self-worth, and mental stability." The final third described treatment goals that focused on building a relationship with the client, such as "the two of you working together and with other health care providers" or "gaining the knowledge of dealing with aspects of another person's mental and psychological background and being able to identify what a person needs and to gain his/her confidence." Some providers identified patient empowerment as a primary goal, such as "the client has a clear idea of where they are heading and will need to work for that" or "helping clients to establish their own goals and a plan that is important to them and then assisting them with the tools needed to meet that goal."

Providers were also asked what "are the major barriers you face in performing your role?" The responses were remarkably similar to those given by mental health care providers, but are not unique given that providers operating in public bureaucracies and seeking services for disenfranchised clients have too few resources, too little time, too many clients, and too much paperwork (Table 3.6). In terms of client-based failures, providers

Table 3.6   Identification of Primary Barriers to Performing Case Management

Barriers to Care	N	%
Lack of Resources/Money/Services	15	34.1
Client Based Failure	7	15.9
Paperwork	6	13.6
Clinician Failure	6	13.6
Too Many Clients/Time	5	11.4
None	5	11.4
Total	44	100.0

targeted "patient non-compliance," or "a lack of follow through," or a lack of self-esteem and social supports. Several providers saw themselves as the primary barrier; one providers said she "needed to acknowledge the needs of my clients." Another felt she had to "get the client to understand my role as it relates to HIV." Providers felt they needed to do more to establish their clients' trust; one targeted her age, "my older HIV clients don't trust me; I have to prove myself," while another said her major barrier was the "clients trusting me because they have been hurt by others."

REDEFINING CASE MANAGEMENT

As noted in the Introduction, changes to the Ryan White authorization made in 2006 have redefined case management. Medicaid requirements have also tightened definitions of what constitutes case management and who may do case management, leading several agencies in the Charlotte TGA to eliminate case management services. I describe these changes and consider the implications of these changes on the ability of service systems to provide comprehensive HIV care.

The Health Resources and Services Administration (HRSA) administers Ryan White funding and has provided concise definitions of case management (Health Services Research Administration, 2008). Referred to as "medical case management," there has been a shift away from the psychosocial rehabilitation described above by case managers to a focus on medication. Medical case management is considered a core service (i.e., part of 75% of core services reimbursable by Ryan White funds for medically necessary services), and in 2006, $135 million was spent on case management. In 2006, case management constituted 33% of state and consortia direct service activities covered under Parts A and B—a considerable amount. To qualify as medical case management, activities must be directly linked to providing, facilitating, or keeping a client in primary medical care. Further, case managers must be part of clinical care teams with direct ties to primary care providers. This has been a hurdle for many HIV agencies, which do not have on-site clinical care services. HRSA still defines core medical case management activities as linking clients to services, coordinating care, and engaging in follow up. Also, case managers can include client-specific advocacy and/or review of utilization of services, although reimbursement for these services is limited. However, greater emphasis is placed on adherence counseling, which I turn to in the next chapter. Non-medical case management, which is still allowed under the 25% of support services funded by Ryan White, "does not involve coordination and follow of medical treatments" (HRSA, 2008). As noted and described in Chapter 2, several agencies had to stop providing case management, as they were not able to meet the criteria of tying case management to clinical care. One agency was in the process of hiring medical staff and reorganizing its case management activities, but it continued to do case management without clinical support or oversight and was closed by HRSA.

Medicaid has also tightened its restrictions over the use of funding for case management, and another leading agency providing case management (that had met HRSA criteria) no longer is able to provide such services (winter 2011). Since Medicaid dollars are administered by the state, I turn to the North Carolina Division of Medical Assistance, 2010 Appropriations Act, Session Law 2010, to illustrate how new regulations are redefining case management. HIV case management is still broadly defined as providing medically necessary services that improve the client's health status and level of functions, and *enhance cost effectiveness*. The revised Medicaid guidelines clearly state that case management must be short term and goal oriented and not long term. Beginning in October 2010, agencies must be certified to offer case management, they must have been offering case management for 3 years, they must have "qualified" case managers and case manager supervisors, and they must have a quality and improvement plan. Qualifications for case managers and supervisors entail increased emphasis on professional preparation, as well as direct work experience; for example, case managers must have 2 years case management experience, with 1 year of HIV case management. Supervisors must have 3 years experience with 2 years of HIV case management (this is in addition to professional degree requirements and supervisory experience). Furthermore, agencies must submit a number of plans (e.g., plans governing confidentiality, non-discrimination, ethics, conflicts of interest, electronic records, transfer, and discharge). They must also submit a supervisor and training plan; a case management orientation plan; a service education plan; a plan for networking with the client's primary care provider; and a plan for tracking case managers' skills, competencies, and knowledge. This is an overwhelming amount of paperwork for what are often small agencies. The large agency referred to previously estimated that the costs of becoming certified were in excess of $10,000 and simply does not have funds for this. The dearth of case management services has been a central focus of concern among advocates and providers in the Charlotte TGA.

The new case management requirements constitute a medicalization of HIV care, with an emphasis on the provision of medically necessary services and narrowed focus on supportive services. Maslow's hierarchy is being reversed. The Medicaid restrictions demonstrate how funding mechanisms increasingly emphasize cost effectiveness and standardized guidelines for care. I will discuss these trends in medical care in Chapter 7; for now, it is sufficient to say that medically necessary care that is cost efficient may not lead to comprehensive care, especially when clients have chronic, multiple heath care conditions that require a broad array of service needs, as well as need for ongoing social supports.

NOTES

1. Examination of the "repeats" allowed me to determine whether providers were consistent in their responses across time; one RN who completed the questionnaire in 4 years of the 5 used almost the exact same words each year in describing her role and treatment goals; only her identification of the barriers to care changed. Other respondents who completed the questionnaire in multiple years also displayed remarkable consistency over time.
2. In order to obtain funding for mental health care, public mental health programs had to meet increased criteria for provider training and certification with an advanced degree—a core requirement for certification as a Community Support Program. Changes in funding and eligibility criteria for HIV case managers are now being implemented by Medicaid restrictions described later in the chapter.
3. These treatment goals are similar to those identified by mental health providers, which ranged from custodial goals to adjustment to autonomy.

4 I Just Don't Feel Like Taking Them
Adherence Counseling and Medical Case Management

INTRODUCTION

This chapter describes an adherence project where health care providers worked collaboratively to develop protocols for intake, medication education, ongoing assessment, and summaries of client outcomes. Part of the impetus for the "Adherence Project," as I refer to it, was federal guidelines for Ryan White that were beginning to redefine case management from a social support to medical model. Several agencies provided supportive counseling, but did not have anyone with a background in adherence counseling. Further, no one was collecting any data on adherence; this project was initiated in order to establish an ongoing evaluation plan for tracking client outcomes and providing for continuous quality improvement. At the time the project was funded in 2002, there was already a great deal of discussion of the CAREWARE data management program required by HRSA. There was broad-based interest in tracking client-level outcomes in order to evaluate HIV care, including medications received and compliance; referrals to both mental health and substance abuse providers, and the ability of these referrals to improve medical outcomes; and interest in the role of clients' (HIV-positive individuals in treatment) own knowledge and behaviors in improving client-level outcomes. In short, adherence was a key research problem defined and driven by the community of HIV providers, rather than academic research that characterizes the majority of the research on HIV treatment adherence.

The Adherence Project first developed a knowledge base to help HIV providers (especially case managers) work with and educate their clients about adherence to HIV medication regimes. The Adherence Project then developed a number of instruments that could be used clinically, as well as for research to assess and track client outcomes. A year after the completion of the first 6 months of the Adherence Project, a large scale interdisciplinary training was held in order to train HIV providers to do adherence counseling with their clients. The project culminated in the development of an adherence manual, which could be distributed to case managers and other providers working with clients to improve their adherence to HIV medications. It was a unique project where I worked collaboratively with health care providers to integrate their clinical work with ongoing evaluation of the outcomes of that work and to disseminate the results of our collaboration to others. One of the core elements of community-based participatory action research is the ability to link practice with research, and this chapter describes a very successful collaborative project. I first begin with a review of the literature on HIV treatment adherence.

HIV DISEASE AND TREATMENT ADHERENCE

HIV/AIDS is a highly infectious disease that is transmitted through bodily fluids and is contracted mainly through unprotected sex, intravenous drug use, or passed from mother to fetus. HIV is a virus that breaks down a person's immune system, or CD4 cells, which is the system that fights disease; the amount of HIV virus in the body is assessed by examining the viral load in the blood (Department of Health and Human Services, 2003). Developed in the mid 1990s, highly active antiretroviral drugs (referred to as HAART) changed the face of HIV disease from a death sentence to a chronic illness for those who could afford the drugs. Antiretroviral drugs function quite simply to reduce the viral load (both by attacking the virus and inhibiting the virus from reproducing), and allow people with HIV disease to live longer and healthier lives. Antiretroviral drugs work by reducing the viral load in the blood and increasing the CD4 count. However, in order to be effective, these drugs must be taken properly.

Antiretroviral drugs have complicated dosing regimes; they must be taken at certain times, with or without food, and have many side effects. In order to reduce the viral load, antiretroviral drugs must be taken correctly 90 to 95% of the time. At the time of the Adherence Project, new HIV drug regimes were being introduced that reduced the number of medications needed to be taken in a day—however, these regimes make adherence even more important, as missing just one dose (i.e., 1 day) has a greater impact. The costs of non-adherence are serious—the virus can mutate and become drug resistant—this is especially likely with the new combinations of non-nucleoside reverse transcriptase inhibitors (NNRTIs or non-nukes) and protease inhibitors. Drug-resistant strains of HIV place the individual at an increased risk of death and also pose a larger public health threat. Consequently, there has been a tremendous amount of research literature reviewing those factors associated with patient adherence to antiretroviral medications (e.g., Catz et al., 2000; Cook et al., 2002; Fogarty et al., 2002; Powell-Cope, White, Henkelman, & Turner, 2003; Safren et al., 2001; Tucker, Burnam, Sherbourne, Kung, & Gifford, 2003; Wainberg & Cournos, 2000). As Demmer (2003) notes, regular assessment of treatment adherence is critical, and health care providers need be involved in the development and evaluation of interventions designed to improve adherence.

As described in Chapter 3, case management is being redefined in terms of medical case management and certainly involves adherence counseling. Medical case management reflects a larger trend toward a medicalized view of HIV treatment, which emphasizes patient non- compliance, rather than a structural view of adherence as a complicated social process that involves enabling or empowering clients and providing them with the knowledge and social supports to comply. What the Adherence Project discovered is similar to Farmer's (2005) observation that patient non-compliance is not the problem, rather it is the failure to develop the patient's sense of trust in their health providers, acceptance of the need for medications, and the ability to continue to take medications in the face of physical side effects and ongoing barriers to care.

The Adherence Project described in this chapter is based on federal redefinitions of case management as medical case management, which requires attention to the medical (as opposed to the social) needs of clients. Specifically, there is a focus on compliance with medical appointments and medications (the operational definition of medical adherence), as well as referrals to social support services (traditional case management includes referrals for housing, mental health, or substance abuse). As codified now into reimbursement formulas for medical case management, case managers must be directly linked to clinical care providers, and we found that interdisciplinary treatment teams were essential to improved adherence. While adherence counseling is clearly a key component of traditional case management, few case managers have the specialized medical knowledge to deal effectively with their clients' barriers to adherence. Reif, Smith, and Golin (2003) describe the adherence-related activities of 94 HIV/AIDS case managers in North Carolina and found that 65% discussed medications with every client; however, they note case managers need more training in medication adherence. With such training, case managers can be more effective in adherence counseling (Shelton, Golin, Smith, Eng, & Kaplan, 2006).

In terms of specific strategies that providers can use, there is some research on provider-based interventions. Brook et al. (2001) report that continuing support from specific health care workers encouraged adherence. Safren et al. (2001) found that motivational interviewing and a problem solving session led to improved adherence for persons with adherence problems. Kalichman et al. (2001) also found that motivational interviewing significantly reduced the number of doses missed. Wainberg and Cournos (2000) report on the effectiveness of mental health counseling. Controlled studies of counseling and education by nurses (Pradier et al., 2002) and pharmacists (Smith, Golen, & Reif, 2004) have found these health care providers to be effective in promoting adherence. Adherence has also associated with good relationships with physicians (Roberts, 2000), although Golin, Smith, and Reif (2004) found that physicians need more training and time to provide adherence counseling to their patients. Likewise, pharmacists often do not have enough time to provide adherence counseling (Smith et al., 2004).

Reif et al. (2003) found that the majority of HIV case managers surveyed in North Carolina did feel adherence counseling was part of their role, although a third did not feel they had adequate training to provide such counseling. Given the dearth of available treatment staff to monitor patient adherence, Broadhead et al. (2002) developed a peer-driven intervention to provide alternative forms of social support for active drug users with HIV infection. Molassiotis, Lopez-Nahas, Chung, and Lam (2003) report on the success of a 3-month patient education model with individualized weekly counseling and follow-up telephone calls. They recommend that clients be supported with individualized management programs, which was the purpose of the adherence counseling model utilized in this study. We referred to the link between the established literature on various techniques to improve adherence and actual client adherence as the "Black Box." Which strategies work with what types of clients; how should an adherence counselor, medical case manager, nurse, or physician decide which strategy is best?

Rather than adopting any one specific adherence strategy, the Adherence Project developed its own strategies after a yearlong experience working with clients referred to the program. The adherence counselors worked collaboratively to enhance their knowledge base and to learn to meet the special challenges posed by clients with various types of obstacles to optimal adherence. They worked with infectious disease doctors and pharmacists to learn the ABC's of HIV medications and obstacles to adherence, and then translated this information for clients. While the adherence counselors in this project worked intensively with HIV-positive individuals to learn to live with HIV and the many problems HAART medications can cause, they also performed many of the duties of a more general case manager and linked their clients to needed social services and supports. More critically, as we will see, the adherence counselors provided a great deal of both tangible and emotional social support, and were mentioned by most clients as the primary health care provider who they could rely on.

THE ADHERENCE PROJECT

The Regional HIV/AIDS Consortium obtained funding to pilot a specialized adherence program for 6 months (November 2001 to June 2002), and funding was continued for another year with additional backing. I served as the evaluator for the project and tracked clients referred to the program during the first year for at least one year. Three individuals were hired from three different counties in the areas served by the Consortium, and each one had different workload expectations. Two of the adherence counselors were nurses, the third a BA social worker; two were White women and one was a Black male (a nurse). One adherence counselor (the social worker) did only adherence counseling full-time, while the two nurses worked part-time as adherence counselors. One nurse (a White female) worked 10 hours per week with adherence clients, and provided ongoing clinical support to a wide variety of clients (not only HIV clients) at her clinic for the remaining 30 hours per week. She did not have her own caseload, but worked intensively with clients needing adherence counseling at that clinical care location. The other nurse (a Black male) provided as much adherence support as was needed, and carried his own caseload of HIV-positive individuals in need of medical supports (generally about 30 to 40 clients at one time). All three found that over the course of the Adherence Project, they gradually took on the role of case manager, as well as adherence counselor; in essence, providing medical case management.

The Adherence Project was an unusual experience, as we all worked intensively together for 2 years and developed integrated clinical and evaluation instruments that provided the adherence counselors with needed clinical information and the evaluator (myself) with needed data for outcome assessment. None of the adherence counselors had any background in adherence, and one of the nurses had no background in HIV disease, so we all had to learn together. We referred to ourselves as the Adherence Team, and spent several months in intensive training on adherence education and outreach before clients were referred to the program. It was a collaborative experience with daily contact via a distribution list I had developed to quickly communicate information we had collected on adherence, and weekly meetings. We learned the newest information about HIV medications and adherence, with several presentations and meetings with pharmacists and intensive reading and sharing of information about HAART medications and adherence. The basic components of HIV patient education include the following (as identified in the Department of Health and Human Services Guidelines, 2003):

- Basic pathophysiology of HIV infection
- Purpose and goals of antiretroviral drugs
- Duration of therapy and administration schedule
- Potential side effects and suggested responses to the side effects
- Concept of resistance and importance of adherence to medication regime
- Potential for drug-drug interactions and important food-drug interactions

Once we had mastered this knowledge base, we continued to meet monthly to develop strategies for improving adherence for the clients referred to the project. In the second year of funding, we developed an Adherence Manual that was used to train new adherence counselors. In the final months of the funding, I worked closely with the adherence counselors to teach them to keep track of their own outcome data.

Let me begin by describing the instruments we used that integrated research tools into ongoing clinical assessments (Appendix B). First, an adherence referral form for use by doctors, nurses, or case managers was developed. Once referred, adherence counselors completed an intake interview that assessed the client's living situation, treatment history, sources of social support, co-occurring health problems, substance use, mental illness, and medical history. If the client had been taking antiretroviral drugs, a 5-day medication recall history was completed. Adherence counselors also completed a 56-item treatment barriers checklist (Catz et al., 2000) to help them determine existing or potential sources of non-adherence. While 56 questions may seem long, in fact the adherence counselors noted that clients' reasons for non-adherence were often not those commonly assessed by shorter scales; they also found that completion of the treatment barriers checklist helped them to know their clients better. Sample items from the treatment barrier included:

- Treatment interferes with time I spend with family and friends.
- I have too many other things to do.
- I don't want to change what I do every day.
- I don't feel comfortable talking to doctors.
- It's hard to plan meals around taking medicine.
- I don't have a good way to keep track of time.

After several preliminary meetings with the client, the adherence counselors completed a treatment plan that could be revised as needed. Following the development of the treatment plan, adherence counselors completed 3-month progress notes to assess adherence, to note any existing problems or concerns, and to describe any changes in the client's living situation. Adherence counselors also noted specific barriers to adherence, as well as clients' strengths relative to adherence.

In terms of my research role as evaluator, I received copies of the intake interview, treatment barriers, medication recall form, and 3-month progress notes, and coded these for data analysis. In addition, I was a member of the Adherence Team, and helped expand clinical knowledge. At regular meetings, we discussed the initial assessments and treatment plans, working collaboratively to solve problems and to modify treatment plans as needed. These meetings were an important component to the Adherence Project's success; as with any team approach, collaborative problem solving is not only instrumentally valuable, it is an important source of social support. Adherence counselors generally worked in isolation and the regular team contact helped them fight the burnout and frustrations detailed in the previous chapter by case managers.

As the Adherence Project moved into its second year, the success of the project necessitated strategies aimed at dissemination. Since it was not practical for most HIV clinics or agencies to each hire an adherence counselor, they asked for multidisciplinary training for case managers to learn to do adherence. This was a 1-day training entitled "HIV Case Manager Adherence Training: A Team Based Approach to Adherence," and included five formal presentations and breakout sessions for participants to develop adherence care plans. A total of 58 HIV case management, mental health, and substance abuse providers attended, and I was one of the presenters. The formal presentations moved beyond basic HIV education to the following topics:

1. Defining Adherence Issues
2. Effectiveness of Team Approaches to Adherence
3. Assessing Patient Readiness: Identifying and Overcoming Barriers
4. Use of Adherence Strategies and Tools: Research Results (my session)
5. Stages of Change to Identify Common Barriers

The development of adherence care plans was based on three different case studies of clients with HIV facing adherence, mental health, and substance abuse problems. Participants were placed into interdisciplinary groups and asked to develop initial assessments. These included responses to the following questions:

1. What are the most pressing clinical issues to address?
2. What does (case subject) see as the pressing issues?
3. What resources does (case subject) have that can help address the situation?
4. Where is (case subject) in the stages of change that can help with these issues?
5. What is your clinical response to the issue given the stage (case subject) is at?

The training and development of adherence care plans was evaluated by participants as highly successful, and in the face of repeated calls for more training, the adherence counselors and I worked to develop a how-to manual to help case managers and HIV providers quickly identify adherence problems, and what types of actions on their part would be most effective in addressing a client's non-adherence. These guidelines were used in subsequent training workshops for HIV case managers and newly hired specialized adherence counselors. The Adherence Manual is a good example of how community-based knowledge can be codified and disseminated, and provides a useful guide for medical case management, as well as for adherence counselors.

The final challenge for the Adherence Project was teaching the adherence counselors to track their own client outcomes. I thought at first this would be fairly simple, as the adherence counselors and I had worked closely together for 2 years on tracking client outcomes and presenting summaries to the Regional HIV Consortium, which managed the funding for the Adherence Project. However, it was the most difficult part of the project. I developed what I thought was a simple client outcome tracking form and had to modify it several times to make it more user-friendly (the final version is shown in Appendix B), and worked with each adherence counselor individually to complete the form at the 3-month scheduled reporting times. I found I had to attend these quarterly meetings several more times before the clinicians were comfortable completing the final outcome reports on their own. Teaching clinicians to think in terms of statistical outcomes (even simple descriptive ones) is probably the most difficult aspect of any community-based research collaboration. I will say more in the concluding chapter, but one major barrier to improved care for HIV clients is the lack of funding for ongoing evaluation and collaborative education. In the following section, I will briefly describe the success of our project in terms of this outcome data, and then I will turn to examine how the adherence counselors were able to attain such an astounding success rate.

ASSESSMENT OF CLIENT OUTCOMES

During the first year of the program, 53 clients were referred for adherence counseling. Of these, 11 were not seen after the initial intake and could not be contacted despite repeated efforts by adherence counselors. Of the 42 seen for continued adherence counseling, five were never placed on HAART and another five died, while two moved out of the service area. Thirty clients were on antiretroviral drugs and received adherence counseling for at least 1 year in order to address problems with adherence.[1] The majority of these clients were male (70%) and African American (83.3%). All clients were receiving Ryan White funding for services. The majority lacked stable social support systems, although they all had case managers (however, as noted above, the adherence counselors often assumed the duties of the case managers).

Adherence was assessed by three measures: client self-report, clinician assessment, and lab work. All three measures of adherence had to concur in adherence for improvement to be noted. That is, if lab work, self-report, and clinician appraisal all indicated improvement in adherence at the 3-month progress report, adherence was assessed as improved. Important to clinician assessment was refill history as assessed by either direct observation (e.g., client brings medications to the clinic, clinician fills prescriptions, or fills pill boxes for the client) or verification by the pharmacist that prescriptions had been refilled, when feasible. Clients were discharged from the program when they had been assessed as fully adherent (no missed doses) for 6 months (through at least two 3-month progress reports); however, clinicians also checked on these clients 6 months after discharge to be sure they were still adherent.

Table 4.1 compares the 6- and 12-month adherence outcomes for these 30 clients. As can be seen, adherence steadily improved for clients with 57% showing improved adherence at the 6-month follow up, and 33% discharged adherent at the 12-month follow up. However, 17% were non-adherent at the 6-month follow up and 10% were still non-adherent at the 12-month follow up. Four clients had been taken off antiretroviral drugs between the

Table 4.1   Six and 12 Month Outcomes for Recipients of Adherence Counseling

	6 Month		12 Month	
	N	%	N	%
Working to Improve Adherence	7	23%	1	3%
Improved Adherence	17	57	12	40
Discharged Adherent	1	3	10	33
Not Adherent	5	17	3	10
Taken off HAART	0	–	4	13%
Totals	30	100%	30	99%

6- and 12-month follow up, due to their lab work indicating some problems or because of co-occurring health problems. We found that there is a need for ongoing and long-term follow up in order to improve adherence, and some clients who were still not adherent at the 12-month follow did eventually show signs of improvement.

What factors contributed to improved adherence? The first step is developed expertise and understanding of HIV adherence and barriers to adherence. As noted above, there is an overwhelming amount of clinically based research on treatment adherence. In order to assist providers, the Department of Health and Human Services provides a user-friendly summary of the scholarly literature and identifies sources of adherence and non-adherence, which we used to develop a clinically based understanding of the existent research literature (these guidelines are updated on a regular basis; I used the 2003 summary to guide the Adherence Project). The Department of Health and Human Services (2003) identifies the major predictors of optimal adherence as:

- Emotional and practical life supports
- Ability to fit medications in daily routine
- Understanding that non-adherence leads to treatment resistance
- Recognition that taking all medication doses as prescribed is critical
- Feeling comfortable taking medication in front of people
- Keeping clinical appointments

In contrast, the following is a summary of the major sources of non-adherence (Department of Health and Human Services, 2003):

- Lack of trust between clinician and client
- Active drug and alcohol use
- Active mental illness or depression
- Lack of patient education and inability of clients to identify medication
- Lack of reliable access to primary medical care or medications
- Side effects

Emotional and social supports are critical resources for adherence. We found that adherence was enhanced when clients express a "will to live" and are ready to work on how to live with the disease. Often, spiritual beliefs are critical to developing a will to live. Another dimension of social support is the critical role a patient has in their family; parenthood was widely recognized to be an important factor in giving clients (especially women) the will to live and to work to improve their health. Once the client is committed to treatment, then the adherence counselor can help educate the client and teach them the importance of taking medications as prescribed and to understand how the medications work. However, too often, patient education proceeds without a thorough understanding of "where the client is at." Readers might turn back to Chapter 2 to see how many clients are in denial about their illness, and hence may not be ready for medication.

Assessment of client adherence and barriers to adherence is the next step for the clinician. We found that using a short-term assessment of medication taken in the recent past (3 to 5 days) and identification of common treatment barriers are helpful in assessing treatment adherence. Having clients bring their medications or medication dairies to clinic visits can be helpful, or checking with the pharmacist to see if prescriptions have been refilled on schedule. Home visits were essential—the clinician can see where medications are kept and assess those factors that prevent optimal adherence. Many clients needed to have the adherence counselor fill their pill boxes on a weekly or biweekly basis. Other clients needed to have the adherence counselor actually fill the prescription for them.

In relation to the Department of Health and Human Services Guidelines, we found that adherence counselors are successful to the degree they develop a good relationship with their clients, especially when the former provide ongoing positive reinforcement and social support. Specifically, adherence counselors:

- Worked to increase clients' understanding of their illness and the need to take medications as prescribed.
- Helped clients to find techniques to cope with the side effects of the medications, and monitor the degree to which side effects result in non-adherence.
- Assisted clients in gaining access to medication through drug assistance programs or other sources, including patient assistance through drug companies.
- Assessed problems with substance use, and discussed with physicians whether medications should be withheld until a client has committed to substance abuse treatment.
- Attended to clients' mental conditions.

Many individuals with HIV disease experience depression and anxiety, and these are major factors to consider in beginning a treatment regime or enhancing adherence. Depression was quite common among clients enrolled in the Adherence Project, and tended to co-occur with other problems related to adherence, as exemplified by AA71, a White woman who had just broken up with her boyfriend, "I feel like nobody cares; I did not forget, I just didn't take them." When she was told that her lab results had worsened, she began taking her medications again, but was still feeling "tired, headachy, and stomach achy," and consequently missed several doses every week. Three months later she got married, and then did not take her medication as "she just did not want to." Despite long-term adherence counseling, the client was still forgetting to take her medications on a regular basis.

Another major barrier to adherence is client denial of the illness (Whetten-Goldstein & Nguyen, 2002). Medication adherence is a daily reminder of the illness, and a common response to any chronic illness is denial. Several of the individuals in the adherence project reported they "did not feel sick enough to be on medications" (PL68, White female and WE63, Black male). Client PL68 "did not have an interest in her treatments, and was bitter over contracting the disease from her husband." HIV disease is highly stigmatizing, and clients are reluctant to disclose their status for fear of discrimination and negative evaluations from family and friends. Consequently, the degree to which a client has accepted their HIV status, and has the support of family and/or friends are critical factors in adherence. Clients are also less likely to take their medications when they are feeling well and believe they do not need medication, or they feel sick and the medications make them feel sicker. For many clients (as we saw in Chapter 2), the illness involves good days and bad days; for example, one Black man in adherence counseling behaved accordingly:

> He knows the schedule; knows how many of each to take; he just decides NOT to take them. Either he feels good and doesn't think he needs them, or he feels bad and doesn't feel like taking them.
>
> (Clinician note on MH50)

This client had a number of problems in the course of the Adherence Project; he was hospitalized for abdominal surgery, and then was burned out of his apartment and went off his medications for a month. His adherence counselor got his prescriptions filled, and helped him to improve both his living situation and family supports. After several months, he was reported to have "made great improvement, but is still missing some doses." The adherence counselor began to fill his pill box weekly and, finally, the client got to the point where he was no longer missing doses. All of the adherence counselors found they had to monitor adherence over a long period of time to help clients learn to live with HIV disease.

Another source of non-adherence is the patient simply forgets, or has trouble fitting the medication into their daily routine. Barfod, Sorensen, Nielsen, Rodkjaer, and Obel (2006) found that "simply forgetting" was the most common reason for missing doses of HIV medication in their cohort study of 840 individuals who either exhibited good treatment adherence or frequently missed doses. Missing doses may be due to work, travel, sleep and eating patterns, being too busy, or other factors relevant to the client's lifestyle. Adherence counselors helped clients find ways to fit medications into their daily routine, and introduced clients to the use of pill boxes, alarms, or various reminder systems to help them remember to take their medications. Eliciting support from family or friends, or other social supports can also help improve adherence in these cases.

COMMUNITY-BASED ADHERENCE STRATEGIES

While the Department of Health and Human Services Guidelines were useful in beginning to think about adherence, we found that the adherence counselors wanted more specific guidance on differential adherence strategies for use with diverse adherence problems. After 2 years of working with clients with adherence problems and ongoing review of the research literature, we decided to codify the practices that seemed to work and to develop guidelines that would help other HIV providers improve treatment adherence. We have found that different strategies work with clients at different stages of "treatment readiness," and the guidelines developed in the Adherence Manual identify critical components of the provider role for each type of client (Scheid, 2007).

More specifically, we found that the role of the adherence counselor changed depending on the major source of the client's non-adherence. When the client is in denial of the illness, generally due to the stigma associated with HIV disease, the clinician needs to work to establish trust and build self-esteem and acceptance of the illness. One of the most damaging consequences of stigma is that individuals internalize the stigmatizing labels, and suffer lower self-esteem and demoralization. The clinician needs to spend time with the client, get to know them, and accept where the client is at. In short, the adherence counselor is a friend, first and foremost.

When the major source of non-adherence is a lack of knowledge about HIV, HIV medications, or side effects, the adherence counselor becomes a teacher, working collaboratively with the client to give them needed information and understanding. Education moves beyond simple biological information about HIV and medications—it critically involves dealing with the patient's perceptions and beliefs about the illness and the efficacy of medication. Whetten-Goldstein and Nguyen (2002) have identified the following as critical to patients' decisions to take medications and to adhere to treatment:

- Trust in the health care system: good experiences with doctors and other providers, feeling that confidentiality is protected, does not believe in conspiracy theory

- Perceived seriousness of the disease
- Perceived susceptibility to future health declines (i.e., it will get better, or worse)
- Perceived benefits of services and treatment
- Perceived value client's support system places on services and treatment
- Perceived ability to use services, to adhere to treatment

The adherence counselor, like any good teacher, must work with the client to alter perceptions, if necessary. Adherence is increased with higher levels of self-esteem, self-efficacy, and when the client feels they have some control. It is very important for the clinician to NOT take on the role of "medication cop."

Even when the client has begun HAART and is compliant, ongoing contact is still necessary. The Adherence Team identified the need for ongoing maintenance versus high level adherence. Maintenance was used for patients who were medically stable on HAART, but needed some form of psychosocial support to maintain their adherence. Most individuals are initially compliant with HAART (for 3 months) and then compliance drops (referred to as pill fatigue). Even when clients had demonstrated adherence, the adherence counselors maintained regular contact with their clients with monthly visits and completion of the 3-month progress notes. They specifically monitored their clients for depression, liver disease, other health problems, and continued or recurring substance abuse. Rather than a teacher, the adherence counselor became a partner, as well a friend.

However, there are clients for whom adherence continues to be problematic. These clients received high level adherence and had at least bimonthly meetings, as well as the 3-month progress notes. These clients often face insurmountable obstacles in their everyday living situations, and consequently, depression and anxiety. Substance abuse is also a key barrier to adherence. The stigma of HIV disease may also limit sources of social support and leave clients isolated. The adherence counselors found that with these most difficult patients, they needed to work to empower clients, and advocate for them to receive other necessary services and supports (e.g., referrals to mental health, substance abuse, or social support groups). It was with the long-term problems with adherence that the adherence counselors became case managers, focused primarily on the provision of social supports and formal services.

Clients were discharged from the Adherence Project once they had been found to be adherent at both the 6-month and 12-month follow ups. In other words, even once found initially adherent, patients were followed up with the 3-month progress notes for a year before being discharged. If during this time adherence again became an issue, the client was then placed on active status and monthly or bimonthly visits began again.

IMPROVING HIV CARE: THE NEED FOR AGGRESSIVE OUTREACH AND SOCIAL SUPPORT

This chapter described a program of specialized adherence counseling and follow up. The project was begun as a pilot and, based on our experience, we developed an adherence manual that has been used in trainings for case managers by local agencies. While the number of clients enrolled in the project was small (we only had funding for three adherence counselors), we found that adherence counseling was successful in that over 70% of the 30 clients who received such counseling demonstrated improved adherence. Of course, some clients with adherence problems were unwilling to meet with an adherence counselor, and these clients are also most likely to "exit" from systems of care. Twenty percent of the clients initially referred for adherence counseling did not continue with counseling after intake, and these clients also were no longer receiving services at the 12-month follow up. This is the most difficult client population to reach, and any provider must work hard to make meaningful contact with clients at the very first visit.

We identified four primary roles performed by the adherence counselor. Adherence counselors were first and foremost "friends" (rather than being "medication cops"); they spent time with clients and helped the clients to accept their illness and deal with the stigma associated with HIV disease. Second, adherence counselors became "teachers" and provided their clients with essential information about HIV disease, HAART medications, and side effects. In the teacher role, adherence counselors worked to distill information from physicians and pharmacists in a language understandable to clients. However, adherence involves more than knowledge—it involves the patients' perceptions and beliefs—and adherence counselors became "partners" with their clients, working to change these perceptions and beliefs as necessary to improve adherence. With those clients dealing with ongoing barriers to adherence (whether mental health, substance abuse, or merely ongoing supports and sustenance issues), the adherence counselors became "advocates" working to link their clients to necessary services.

Because so many clients are non-compliant with appointments, as well as medication, the most important factor in the success of our adherence program was that counselors went to clients' homes rather than relying on office-based visits. Clinic appointments can place the provider in a more powerful position relative to the client and may mitigate the feeling of trust that is critical to adherence. Home visits also allow the adherence counselor to see where medications are kept and to assess factors that contribute to non-adherence. The ultimate goal is client empowerment, where clients take ownership of their illness and responsibility for their improved health. The adherence counselor's difficult job is not merely to improve medication compliance, but to get clients to this final stage.

We found that the ultimate key to the success of our program was developing an open, trusting relationship with clients and providing positive (not negative) reinforcement. Crucial to adherence is acceptance of the illness, understanding of the role of medications, and a positive sense that taking medication will help. Adherence counselors helped clients gain that sense of mastery and also helped them cope with the stigma of HIV disease. Adherence counselors were also an important source of social support for clients that had very few other resources. Obviously, adherence counseling is not a quick fix, but adherence is not simply a medical issue. Instead, adherence involves the full spectrum of an individual's life and belief system, and changing these to improve adherence will take more than one patient education session. Adherence counseling does work and should be a critical component to HIV disease management, but there is a need for long-term follow up and continued patient education in order to fully address non-adherence. Because of the need for continued support, adherence counseling should be a key component to medical case management and team-based approaches. In the next chapter, we build on the adherence training described in this chapter to consider the role of interdisciplinary cross-training in enhancing the ability of HIV case managers to provide integrated HIV care.

NOTE

1. Other studies of adherence interventions have also been based on a relatively small number of study participants. Molassiotis et al. (2003) report on a pilot study in a group of six non-adherent men. Shelton et al. (2006) studied 16 case managers who were trained and then each worked with 1 to 4 clients in their study of adherence counseling. The Adherence Project described in this chapter is valuable in that strategies were developed for different types of adherence problems. Specific strategies would need to be evaluated in a more controlled study with a larger number of participants, although it is very difficult to study the effect of the clinician-patient relationship in a clinical study. One factor clearly needing a more controlled assessment was our experience that home visits were essential.

5 Finding Common Ground
Professional Cross-Training for Collaborative Systems of Care

INTRODUCTION

This chapter examines professional cross-training as one strategy to meet the multiple needs of people living with HIV/AIDS. Cross-training is a mechanism to coordinate care at the client level, where providers (and sometimes clients) receive training in service systems outside of their primary service involvement, as well as training in cultural competence. Another strategy for client-level integration is the use of multidisciplinary treatment teams, where providers with different areas of expertise meet and plan for coordinated treatment for their clients. Both cross-training and multidisciplinary treatment teams seek collaborative models of care that revolve around the specific needs of a given client. This chapter focuses on cross-training, and is based on the experience of a group of providers who worked together to develop a curriculum for cross-training (referred to as the Common Ground), and who implemented this cross-training over the course of several years and subsequently trained new faculty to conduct cross-training. This chapter is arguably the most applied in the book, in that it builds on years of collaborative experience doing cross-trainings by providers and educators to provide a "how-to" model for cross-training. Consequently, this chapter will be useful to those who are actually seeking to implement cross-training, or for those who want to increase the effectiveness of multidisciplinary treatment teams.

HIV clients need a comprehensive array of services, as well as continuity of care. However, HIV, substance abuse, and mental health services are delivered within independent service systems and organizations (Meyerson & Scofield, 1999). Providers generally have expertise in one, perhaps two, areas of disability and illness—HIV/AIDS, mental health, or substance abuse. Because of the co-occurrence of mental health and substance abuse, many mental health care providers do have training in substance abuse, although the treatment orientations differ (Burton et al., 2001). However, mental health and substance abuse providers often lack basic training in HIV/AIDS, and many are not adequately trained to take sexual or drug-use risk histories, nor are they able to assess HIV risk (Behavioral Social Science and Prevention Research

Area Review Panel, 1996; Carey, Weinhardt, & Carey, 1995; Knox, 1989; Walkup, Satriano, Hansell, & Olfson, 1998). Consequently, providers are not able to refer their clients to appropriate services.

As we saw in Chapter 2, individuals with a positive HIV diagnosis are also at risk for mental health problems (Batki, 1990; Crystal & Schlosser, 1999; Simoni & Ng, 2000), including depression and anxiety. In addition to anxiety and depression following a positive HIV diagnosis, HIV sero-positivity strains social relationships and supports, and results in a great deal of stress in life due to changes in work status and the experience of acute illnesses and adherence to complicated medication regimes. Many individuals consider HIV/AIDS to be a death sentence, and are at higher risk for suicide (Crystal & Schlosser, 1999). HIV/AIDS providers may have some background in either substance abuse or mental health, but many HIV/AIDS providers are not adequately trained to recognize mental health symptoms or to elicit information about their patients' mental health status, and may not be aware of the mental health services available to their clients. Because of heavy caseloads and multiple demands, providers often work in isolation and have limited connections to other types of treatment providers and resources. Consequently, there is a need to extend and integrate providers' knowledge about the interrelationships of HIV, mental health, and substance abuse, and providers need further training to recognize and proactively deal with their clients' substance abuse and/or mental health problems.

CROSS-TRAINING

Federal agencies (including SAMHSA, the CDC, and HRSA) have developed a number of initiatives based on cross-training, where individuals from different disciplines are brought together and educated about how to integrate services. These cross-trainings have focused on HIV/AIDS and substance abuse, and generally target minority populations. Often, cross-training is directed to increasing the cultural competence of providers. SAMHSA's Center for Substance Abuse Treatment (CSAT) has developed a number of tools and treatment protocols to deal with both substance abuse and risk for HIV, and in 1993, joined with the CDC to develop a cross-training initiative. In 1998, HRSA joined in these collaborative efforts to provide training resources (Quander, 2000). A 2-day training initiative was developed with diverse modules that could be adapted to different problems and populations. In addition, SAMHSA has promoted specialized cross-training modules and also developed a curriculum to prepare individuals to become trainers able to conduct regular cross-training workshops. However, in the Charlotte area, cross-training developed from the ground up with the growing awareness that providers needed training beyond their own areas of specialization because of the co-occurring nature of their clients' illnesses.

Providers' perceptions were supported by a variety of needs assessments conducted by various agencies who subsequently became involved in cross-training (see below). Specifically, there was consensus that:

- Existing services were not meeting the needs of HIV/AIDS consumers who were also diagnosed with substance abuse and/or mental health disorders.
- Services and professional competencies among HIV/AIDS, SA, and MH providers needed to be integrated to effectively improve treatment outcomes and the quality of life of multiply diagnosed consumers.
- Provider competencies needed to be enhanced.
- Cross-training was needed so that providers in different service areas could come together and learn about each other's disciplines, combine professional competencies, and create mutually reinforcing services and care practices.

The initial Common Ground trainings were sponsored by the Charlotte Area Health Education Center (AHEC), largely through the efforts of the Director of Mental Health Education. A core faculty, consisting of HIV and mental health providers, as well as consumers, sponsored a number of continuing education sessions for local agencies beginning in 1996. The health department also actively promoted cross-training, and made support for the Common Ground cross-training a key feature of its plan to integrate HIV, MH, and SA services (see Chapter 6). However, it was the Charlotte Regional HIV/AIDS Consortium (serving a 13-county region in North and South Carolina) that sponsored and supported the Common Ground cross-training project. Training and continuing education of HIV providers and case managers was part of the mission of the Charlotte Regional HIV/AIDS Consortium, which also had SAMHSA funding that helped it to support cross-training for not only HIV case managers, but mental health and substance abuse providers.

The Common Ground faculty initially included qualified HIV/AIDS trainers who had been directors of education at AIDS service organizations. The majority also had expertise in substance abuse treatment and credentials as substance abuse counselors and supervisors, or were licensed clinical social workers in private practice. The faculty grew to include substance abuse and mental health care providers, and consumers of HIV/AIDS, SA, and MH services. Minority providers and consumers were actively recruited and involved in trainings and as faculty. Team teaching allowed faculty to focus on their areas of special expertise and build on each other's knowledge.

The original faculty organized within AHEC built on their years of experience and worked hard to codify a curriculum that preserved the experiential and grounds up nature of the original cross-trainings. The cross-training faculty came from diverse backgrounds, had different kinds of educational credentials, served different clients, and worked in different organizations.

Their treatment ideologies (or philosophies) were quite different (see Chapter 3). Treatment ideology is the complex set of beliefs that healthcare providers hold about health, illness, and treatment (Scheid, 1994). These beliefs consist of specific theories about the etiology of illness, the role of the patient or client, and the validity or efficacy of various treatments (see Abbott, 1992; Eaton et al., 1990; Strauss et al., 1964). Such ideologies guide the treatment decisions and behaviors of providers—they tell the provider what to do and how to do it. As has been well established, practical work experiences can shape treatment philosophies (Benner, 1984), and the cross-training faculty believed firmly that the only way to change fixed treatment preferences and disciplinary isolation was experiential learning.

Experiential learning integrates concrete learning with reflective observations about the learning experience (Cantor, 1995). Such learning is flexible and highly interactive with a great deal of personal involvement (Rogers, 1969). As such, the Common Ground training allows for convergence across traditional professional boundaries, and helps providers develop new fundamental principles of care; consequently, changing their treatment ideologies. Case simulations and role-playing allow providers to recreate their treatment ideologies and, hence, develop standards for care that will promote the development of integrated care plans.

The goal is that cross-training can integrate the treatment practices of HIV/AIDS, SA, and MH providers by promoting effective communication and coordination, as well as developing convergences across the three disciplines. Special emphasis was placed on cultural competence and on training providers who serve women and African Americans, with a recent concern to address the needs of Hispanic clients. An innovative feature of Common Ground was its inclusion of consumers and volunteers as both faculty and training participants. The assumption is that consumer/client involvement enhances the providers' experience and allows for client-centered care. The cross-training sessions also assist providers by introducing new types of solutions and ways of thinking about overcoming disciplinary boundaries and medicalized, individualized care. Consequently, the hope is that with cross-training, providers will feel greater professional empowerment, more satisfaction, and experience lower levels of psychological burnout. Likewise, consumers undergoing cross-training will also gain needed insight into the management of their multiple health problems, feel empowered, and experience greater satisfaction with their care. Additionally, providers and consumers will gain insight into, and respect for, each other's experiences and expectations leading to better communication. Consumers can go on to serve as peer counselors and will be able to assist other consumers in gaining insight into the management of their care (see Chapter 2). The anticipated result is a higher degree of patient-centered holistic care, as well as higher quality care across diverse settings and over time.

THE COMMON GROUND MODEL

The Common Ground model includes three levels of training:

Level I: Building Common Ground

This establishes a shared knowledge base among HIV, SA, and MH providers using targeted conferences and in-house training seminars sponsored by agencies. The learning objectives for Level I include:

- Developing a basic understanding of current HIV/AIDS, SA, and MH issues and practices.
- Developing an appreciation for the roles of service providers in providing treatment and care, which includes educating consumers about HAART and strategies for treatment adherence.
- Introducing strategies to overcome various barriers clients face in seeking services and treatment.
- Identifying and discussing issues and conflicts among local cultural, racial, and ethnic minorities affected by HIV/AIDS.

Level II: Bridging Clinical Gaps

Level II is a highly structured, dynamic, and interactive training experience. The objective is to blend a variety of perspectives and disciplines to develop coherent strategies that use the strengths of each perspective. Level II focuses on relationship building and overcoming barriers, and uses role-playing to enable participants to understand other perspectives. Participants are provided with readings that focus on the multiple problems of populations at risk for HIV/AIDS. Informational discussion sessions (including a pharmacy update) are followed by three role-playing sessions. The role-playing sessions involve a facilitator and co-facilitator and a variety of client roles that represent hard-to-reach populations (e.g., a Spanish-speaking woman, a homeless person with mental illness, a young gay White man who is into club drugs, a woman newly released from prison who is in an abusive relationship). The role-playing sessions occur within the context of a support group for clients, and participants stay in the same role for all three sessions and experience the barriers to care faced by these clients. After the role-playing, a debriefing session is held and participants share how each experienced their own and others' roles. These role-playing sessions allow providers to gain an in-depth understanding of their clients' lives. The learning objectives for Level II include:

- Developing an emotional understanding of the ways HIV/AIDS, SA, and MH problems impact people over time.

- Developing a greater appreciation for the unique ways people cope with trauma and crisis.
- Confronting a trauma-rich setting without developing vicarious trauma.
- Supporting consumers and providers.

Level III: Care Planning

The focus of Level III is on developing assessment and treatment plans that meet the multiple needs of triply diagnosed clients and are culturally sensitive. Level III involves a workshop organized around case presentations and group case consultation with the goal being the development of integrated treatment plans. The experiential learning model is organized around the three cases introduced in Level II. A working team role-plays a care planning session with two observer teams attending to the process with feedback. Observer teams take notes through four "lenses": client involvement, culture, gender, and supportive relationships. The outcome is a care plan for each client that captures the issues uppermost for that client. Consequently, the ultimate goal of Level III training is client-centered care that takes into account the multiple needs of clients with HIV/MH/SA problems. The specific objectives of Level III include:

- Developing integrated assessment and treatment plans.
- Developing intervention strategies.
- Understanding of and respect for the clients' needs and preferences for care.
- Developing tools for dealing with difficult ethical decisions.

Because the learning is experiential, the specific Common Ground curriculum varied each time it was offered. A team of four to five faculty (the Common Ground faculty consisted of 10 to 15 members who met at least twice a year to plan for upcoming cross-trainings) organized and conducted each cross-training. I was a member of the faculty (having joined in 2000) and I served as faculty for all cross-trainings held over the course of 5 years, and then spear-headed an effort to extend the Common Ground faculty by conducting a cross-training to train more faculty in 2005, which built on both the Common Ground curriculum and the SAMHSA materials for Cross-Training for Collaborative Systems of Prevention, Treatment, and Care (Center for Substance Abuse Treatment, 2007). Faculty were selected who represented the diverse service sector areas of HIV, mental health, and substance abuse at a minimum, with other service sectors represented as necessitated by the target audience (e.g., the sample curriculum that follows targeted the criminal justice system and the need for housing for the homeless). Cross-training workshops were held over 2 days, although we did develop a 1-day module for individuals who had already completed Level I objectives by obtaining basic information on diverse service systems (HIV 101, Mental Health 101,

Substance Abuse 101). The learning objectives and outcomes for a 2-day workshop are outlined in the next section and can serve as a model for other communities seeking guidance on cross-training.

BUILDING CONNECTIONS: PROFESSIONAL CROSS-TRAINING FOR COLLABORATIVE SYSTEMS

The following sections provide a summary of the cross-training modules we developed and can be adopted for use by other groups or communities seeking to implement cross-training in their communities. The following description was used to advertise the cross-training in promotional materials:

> The Building Connections Cross-Training is offered over 2 days and focuses on care planning and prevention for persons at risk for HIV/AIDS with co-occurring mental health and/or substance abuse problems. These individuals are often homeless or have a need for supportive housing and may have encounters with the criminal justice system. The Cross-Training is designed to bring together providers from diverse service systems and enable them to build connections, which will lead to more coordinated treatment for persons in need of multiple services. The target audience is individuals providing services or care in the HIV/AIDS, Substance Abuse, Mental Health, Criminal Justice, and Homeless Service sectors.

Overall Objectives

- Identify existing barriers to comprehensive, coordinated services and develop strategies for change.
- Improve cross-disciplinary communication and coordination of client care.
- Identify practical and recovery related needs of those with multiple problems and locate helpful resources.
- Increase personal and professional awareness of the problems faced by persons with HIV, substance abuse, and mental health problems.

Schedule of Activities

Day 1, Level I: Making the Connection
  8:30–9:30: Introductions and Profile of the Consumer
  9:30–10:00: Brainstorming to Identify Potential Challenges Faced (Since folks will be walking around, they can incorporate break into this time slot as they wish.)
  10:15–11:00: Small Group Activity with Leading Questions
  11:00–12:00: Groups Report Out and Have a Conversation—"What does it all mean?"
  12:00–1:00: Lunch Break

1:00–2:30: Short Informational Sessions, HIV, MH, SA (Speakers limited to 20 minutes each, end with time for participants to contribute their own knowledge base, develop list of barriers to integrated treatment.)

2:30–2:45: Break

3:00–4:30: What Else Does the Client Need? (What's new in Housing options, Social Services, Criminal Justice. Session to end with questions participants felt needed to be addressed on Day 2.)

Day 2, AM; Level II: Bridging Service System Gaps

8:30–9:00: Walk About

9:00–10:15: Developing Multidisciplinary Collaborations

10:15–11:00: Break

11:00–12:00: Establishing Memorandum of Agreement, Protecting Client Confidentiality, Code of Ethics (SAMHSA guidelines)

12:00–1:00: Lunch

Day 2, PM; Level III: Strategic Development and Care Planning

1:00–2:30: Client Assessment and Treatment Protocols

2:30–3:00: Break

3–4:30: Bringing It All Together

Level I: Making the Connection

These information-based sessions establish a shared knowledge base among providers working in diverse systems of care.

Objectives:

1. Develop a basic understanding of current issues and practices within each system sector that impacts client care, treatment, and prevention.
2. Develop an appreciation of the roles of diverse service providers in providing care, treatment, and prevention.
3. Develop an understanding of the need for collaborative systems of care.

Outcomes:

1. Increased understanding and comfort in working with problems not included in one's own professional training.
2. Increased awareness of the need to screen for other disorders and increased screening for diverse risk factors.
3. Appreciation for problems faced by providers working in other system sectors.

Activities:

I. Defining the Client: Facilitators will each contribute to a client monologue, beginning with a statement of HIV-positive status, moving to a consideration of mental health issues, then substance abuse problems. Participants will brainstorm the potential challenges facing clients with co-occurring problems using newsprint to write down one challenge they recognize.

II. Client profiles will be introduced to groups of 4–5. Each facilitator will act as one of the profiled clients and work with the group to identify barriers to treatment via the leading questions exercise (developed by Joanne Jenkins, Common Ground faculty).

   a. Participants to share one or two questions they have about the client.
   b. Participants identify the connecting threads/themes in their questions.
   c. Participants will discuss the best ways to answer the questions.

III. Each group reports what the themes are based on the previous exercise—"What does it all mean?"

IV. Short Information Sessions Addressing HIV, MH, and SA: What are existing resources for treatment of clients with co-occurring problems? What is new in each area in terms of treatment options? Each facilitator takes 15–20 minutes for presentation of information with participants generating a list of what is new in their domain/agency/field and how they provide care to clients in their systems, as well as describing how they currently respond to clients with diverse needs.

V. What Else Does the Client Need? (Address this with guest speakers; could be clients or providers).

   a. Housing
   b. Subsistence, Income, Medications
   c. Social Support
   d. Involvement in the Criminal Justice System

Have participants develop a list of priorities to meet the needs of the client they discussed in the morning session (i.e., first this client needs, then they need . . .). Have participants share their priorities and determine to what degree each area of specialization/treatment sector influenced how they prioritized the client's needs. Faculty can start a discussion of Maslow's hierarchy of needs (e.g., clients are less concerned with health status than with meeting daily subsistence needs, such as housing, food, or income, and substance use may well be a way to deal with the stress of having unmet basic needs).

Level II: Bridging Service System Gaps

Stage II consists of simulated experiences and role-playing that allow providers to gain an experiential understanding of the barriers faced by persons with multiple problems.

Objectives:

1. Experience the barriers faced by persons needing services from diverse systems.

2. Develop an empathetic understanding of the ways that multiple problems impact people over time and develop respect for the unique ways people cope with trauma and crisis.
3. Understand the need for collaborative systems of care.

Outcomes:

1. Increased empathy for clients and their challenges.
2. Increased understanding of challenges faced by providers in diverse systems.
3. Increased ability to identify other providers available in diverse systems.

Activities:

I. Walk About Exercise (developed by Joanne Jenkins, Common Ground faculty).

   a. Ask participants to walk around the room in any direction. Ask them to stop and close their eyes. Say, "You are having lots of diarrhea, which makes you think you may have HIV. How do you feel?" Faculty to gather responses and record on a flip chart.
   b. Ask participants to open their eyes and walk around the room. Stop. "You are now at the testing center. You have just been told that you are HIV-positive. How does this make you feel?" Record responses on a flip chart.
   c. Ask participants to continue walking around the room. Stop. "You have now lived with HIV for 2 years and your health is deteriorating. Your symptoms are full blown. Your family is ashamed and won't talk about your illness with you, and you haven't told any of your friends. How does that make you feel?" Record responses on a flip chart.
   d. Ask participants to walk in a circle around one person who is "HIV-positive." Stop. "Show how you are feeling toward this person with your body. What are you thinking?" Then ask the person in the center, "How are you feeling?"

Faculty work to establish that the point of this last step is to show how providers generally do not want to touch their clients. The professional model is one of detachment; we need to move beyond the clinician versus client role to collaborative care where the client is a partner.

II. Establishing Multidisciplinary Collaborative Networks (Center for Substance Abuse Treatment, 2007). This is a small group exercise where participants identify:

   a. The Characteristics of a Collaborative Network
   b. The Challenges Faced in Establishing Collaborative Networks
   c. Specific Strategies to Overcome the Challenges Identified

The exercise ends with a discussion of the stages of collaboration where providers move from mere co-existence (with each provider in their own domain or silo) to co-ownership. Participants then identify specific strategies they will use to achieve better levels of coordination.

Level III: Strategic Development and Care Planning

The focus of the third stage is to develop assessment and treatment plans that meet the multiple needs of clients and are culturally sensitive, and to also develop strategies for system change.

Objectives:

1. Development of understanding of, and respect for, clients' needs and preferences for care.
2. Development of integrated assessment, prevention, and treatment plans.
3. Development of strategies for collaboration and assessing readiness for change and identification of tools for dealing with system barriers.

Outcomes:

1. Increased confidence in designing treatment plans.
2. Ability to develop strategies that meet clients' unique needs.
3. Increased confidence in interacting with providers in other service systems on behalf of the client, and overcoming system barriers.

Activities:

I. Integrated Assessment and Treatment Protocol: Groups to return to their client (with a facilitator acting as the client, as in day 1). Complete an assessment and develop a treatment protocol for that client using SAMHSA assessment/treatment protocol.

II. Bring It Together: Each group presents their assessment and treatment plan, which will be critiqued by the entire group.

ASSESSMENT OF THE COMMON GROUND CURRICULUM

The Common Ground faculty, with support from the Regional HIV/AIDS Consortium, not only sponsored a number of cross-trainings (including a final session dedicated to training individuals to go on and conduct their own cross-trainings) but sought funding to implement and evaluate the Common Ground curriculum. While ultimately not funded, cross-trainings were systematically evaluated, qualitative data was collected from participants and faculty, and debriefings were held. Participants in the cross-training from which this data is drawn include providers and consumers: seven were Black women, three were White women, two were Black men, and three were White men.[1] Four of the Black women (all consumers) came from a Peer Education project elsewhere in the state, with the intention of using the cross-training to help them with that project. The others came from a broad mix of service agencies for HIV, mental health, and substance abuse, and many were case managers, with client loads averaging 21 (although one provider in a rural county had 38 HIV clients). In terms of their evaluation of the Common Ground training, 77% were very satisfied; 77% would recommend it to others; 85% would recommend it to their colleagues; 77% felt the objectives were clear and were largely met; and 92% found the subject matter well organized and suitable. All of the participants valued the information they got on accessing resources for their clients. They appreciated "learning about strategies for hard-to-manage clients." Participants especially liked the interactive sessions, and felt they had developed not only more empathy for their clients, but for providers in other sectors. Networking (and provider social support) was clearly an important outcome. The cross-training was fun, and providers felt renewed energy and enthusiasm for their work. The other cross-trainings also had consistently high evaluations, with good suggestions for revisions to the curriculum, which are reflected in the Common Ground model described above.

However, the evaluations of the cross-training workshop do not assess the overall impact of the cross-training on providers' actual treatment choices or practices. I will try to give the reader some insight into how the Common Ground experience had changed providers' thinking about treatment by sharing the client profiles introduced in Level I, around which care plans were developed in Level III. The discussion of the clients and the development of care plans allow us to see into providers' logics in use. As noted above, we began by having each faculty member be the client profiled, and we rehearsed our roles and developed an extended monologue around the details of each client. We then played the client in the initial group meeting where questions were asked about each client, which then led to the leading questions exercise. The leading questions were then used to establish collaborative treatment plans, which were critiqued by the entire group at the end of the cross-training. I share three client profiles and the questions that emerged from the leading questions exercise, as well as preliminary treatment plans, in order for the reader to see how disciplinary barriers can indeed be overcome with cross-training.

Client Profile 1: You are a White female, 52 years old, and you have been separated from your husband for 2 years after you learned of an affair. You have been afraid to have an HIV test, but your women's support group convinced you, and your doctor thought it was a good idea.

The client (faculty in role-play) presented herself as emotionally detached and bitter; she is concerned about her work and home. She is also still resistant to the idea of testing, saying she has not experienced any symptoms of HIV/AIDS. Further, she is fearful of the testing itself, asking, "How confidential is the testing procedure?" "How are the results presented?" The providers responded that this client needed education about the facts of HIV/AIDS, and she needed a thorough mental health and social support assessment. Specifically, a full assessment of the client's history and her emotional, spiritual, and ongoing social supports was needed. The client needed to address the future: What were her plans? Did she hope for reconciliation? Was she in a safe place? Did she have financial stability (now and going into old age)?

Client Profile 2: You are a 35-year-old, college-educated, Puerto Rican bisexual male who has been HIV-positive for 8 years. You visit NYC regularly for the relative anonymity of sex and drugs away from your girlfriend, family, and friends, who do not know of your sexual orientation, drug use, or HIV status. You refuse to take any medications, as you believe they are harmful to your body.

The client (faculty in role-play) presented himself as confrontational: "Why do I have to do this?" "What can it do for me?" "Is this confidential?" He became more conciliatory, asking, "Are there others like me?" "Who do I have tell my status to?"

The providers sought to gain insight into his behavior, asking him, "What triggers your trips to NYC? What are you getting?" "Are you using protection?" "Are your partners positive or negative?" "What is your drug of choice?" Questions then moved to the client's health status: "How do you feel?" "Why no medications?" "What other care do you receive (alternative or medical)?" "Have you ever had a mental health assessment?" "Do you fear death?" The providers' preliminary treatment plan focused more directly on the client's supports and ties with family and friends: "Who are your main sources of social support; who do you turn to when you need to talk?" "What will happen if you tell your girlfriend, family, and friends about your sexual orientation, drug use, or HIV status?" Providers felt this client needed to be a full partner in any treatment plan, and that he had to make the decision to commit to making lifestyle changes before much could be done for him.

Client Profile 3: You are a 32-year-old Black woman with a history of psychotic episodes. You live in a boarding house and freely engage in unprotected sex with the other residents.

The client (faculty in role-play) presented herself as isolated and lonely: "Will someone love me?" "How do I stop?" "Can I get my kids back?" "Where else can I live?" Providers again stressed the need for patient education and information about HIV and STDs, the need for testing, and to help the client understand her own risk behavior and methods for HIV prevention (e.g., use of a condom). A preliminary treatment plan included a full mental health assessment, taking a substance abuse and medication history, looking into possible domestic violence and any criminal history, as well as history of psychiatric hospitalizations. The plan included finding the client alternative housing and linking her to both social support groups and spiritual support sources.

INTEGRATED CARE AND STRATEGIES FOR
BUILDING COLLABORATIVE NETWORKS

While increasing collaboration among providers is difficult, the Common Ground model described above is based on years of collaboration among providers in diverse settings and can serve as a model, saving others seeking to implement cross-training (or even just improve multidisciplinary communication) a great deal of time. In our final wrap up session in this cross-training, providers and faculty identified the following components of integrated treatment. First, integrated treatment must meet the client's basic needs. Providers have to be "where the client is at . . . they can't just try to fix the client." This means establishing trust and doing what the client wants, not necessarily what the provider thinks is best. Second, providers have to serve as advocates for their clients, even when no one "wants" a particular client (we also saw this in Chapter 3 in describing the role of case managers, as well as in Chapter 4). The role of the provider was to move progressively from that of a facilitator (who helps her clients meet their basic needs) to that of an enabler who empowers clients. This is similar to the role of adherence counselors, and can certainly serve as a model for those currently engaged in medical case management. However, cross-training goes beyond case management to emphasize collaboration between providers, rather than only addressing the client/provider relationship. Third, in order to provide for integrated care, providers must work together to understand and meet the diverse needs of their clients.

Following the exercise outlined in Level II of the Common Ground curriculum, participants identified the characteristics of a collaborative network, and the barriers to achieving such networks (be they through cross-training or multidisciplinary treatment teams). The characteristics of a collaborative network are: commitment (people coming to the table), representative (everyone has to be at the table), and agreement on both roles and goals. In terms of agreement on roles and goals, following the recommendations of Rier and Indyk (2006), each type of provider and consumer must be recognized for their expertise and everyone must acknowledge that all types of expertise are valuable. The obstacles to these collaborative networks are well known, and were identified by participants in the cross-trainings when they were asked to describe the challenges faced in establishing collaborative networks. The obstacles to commitment include a lack of time, hidden agendas about why a provider is at the table, and unresolved conflicts between providers. The obstacles to representation include a lack of availability, who decides who can come to the table, and unequal status among those at the table (hierarchy). Agreement on roles and goals is limited by the use of language exclusive to one's own professional background or domain, different priorities, and domain disputes.

Domain disputes are at the heart of these obstacles to reform—they produce unresolved conflict and are reflected in hierarchical interactions.

While the cross-training educated providers about the need for collaboration, they were "unsure how to set up pathways for such communication." Most importantly, provider cross-trainings cannot really overcome system-level barriers to care, such as the lack of shared assessment tools, or scarce resources that limit collaborative efforts. Agencies are often in competition for scarce funding, especially grant monies. Participants in the cross-trainings themselves recognize these barriers, and all agreed that market-driven health care and categorical funding mechanisms worked to undermine any efforts to integrate HIV care. They agreed that providers need to not only advocate for their clients, but for changes in the system. In the following chapter, we focus more directly on system fragmentation.

NOTE

1. I used the 2005 Common Ground cross-training curriculum, as that was the last one we developed and the one where the curriculum was felt to be the best. This cross-training also followed our training of other faculty, and utilized their input in the development of the Common Ground curriculum.

6   Integrating Systems of Care
for Multiply Diagnosed
HIV/AIDS Clients

INTRODUCTION

HIV disease is no longer a death sentence; it has become a chronic illness. Chronic health care systems require a diverse array of both medical and social support services. This is especially true of HIV disease, which often involves physical health care, mental health care, and substance abuse treatment, as well as the provision of basic necessities, such as housing and income, to individuals who are socially marginalized. In order to provide for wholistic care, these diverse systems need to be integrated. Klinkenberg and Sacks (2004) have argued that treatment programs for multiply diagnosed HIV-positive individuals must provide some level of integrated care to be effective. Successful integration of HIV care systems will have important lessons for communities seeking to integrate health care services for other chronic care populations, as well as the elderly.

At the same time that the number of individuals with chronic care needs has increased, the health care sector has undergone profound organizational change in response to wider social forces promoting the corporatization and commodification of health care (Light, 1997; Relman, 1980; Scheid, 2003; Scott, Ruef, Mendel, & Caronna, 2000). Managed care has been the organizational response in the U.S. to these larger forces, and has been propelled by an overriding concern to control costs (Wholey & Burnes, 2000). With managed care, decisions to reimburse health services are based on external determinations of medical necessity. A health condition must have a valid medical diagnosis, result in impaired functioning, and treatment must be effective and justified by research to be efficacious. Treatment is expected to result in some measurable improvement, if not ultimately in the cure. Managed care is obviously designed for acute health problems that meet the condition of medical necessity (Schlesinger & Mechanic, 1993); it is also both cause and consequence of forces promoting medicalization (Conrad, 2007). Managed care imposes a medical model on care systems; however, sociologists have argued that the diagnostic disease model is not appropriate for the care of chronic illnesses (Kleinman, 1988; Mechanic, 1995; Strauss, Fagerhaugh, Suczek, & Wiener, 1985) because it focuses exclusively on a given medical condition and its treatment.

While wholistic care for chronic care conditions such as HIV disease requires system-level integration of diverse services and supports, integration by itself can be a "panacea"—it is offered as the "cure" without a realistic understanding that the integration of inadequate and underfunded systems of care will not improve health care (Scheid, 2004a). In this chapter, I discuss a project that was funded to develop a plan to integrate multiple chronic care systems (HIV disease, mental health, and substance abuse) for minority clients. The Integration Project (as I will refer to it) moved beyond client-based integration and provider collaboration to the larger task of trying to integrate diverse systems of care at the systems level. In addition to a focus on integration, this chapter describes efforts to develop community-based coalitions, which are an important mechanism for system integration, as well as health care reform. I will proceed by first presenting the theoretical case for integration (i.e., coordination of care and organizational efficiencies), and examining various ways that systems can be integrated.

HEALTH CARE INTEGRATION AND FRAGMENTATION

Service system integration is defined in terms of interorganizational relationships or network ties between agencies in a given sector. Interorganizational relationships help organizations manage their agencies' interdependencies (Longest, 1990). More critically for chronic care populations, integration enables individuals with diverse service needs to access needed services. Health care integration can occur at various levels: the client level with the coordination of clinical care via case management as described in Chapters 3 and 4, the provider level with cross-training as described in Chapter 5, or the organizational level with HMOs and other "one-stop shop" models of care. In addition, there are many different types of vertical or horizontal integration between organizational units (such as networks of hospitals and community agencies) and, finally, systems themselves can be integrated with some kind of overriding authority over all the organizations in a given sector.

Most studies of integration focus on organizational integration, often with the hospital as the center of control. An example is Charns (1997), who describes four stages to the development of healthcare integrated systems. There is first competition and little interdependence among hospitals. A system of pooled interdependencies results in horizontal integration, which is followed by sequential interdependencies (vertical integration). The final stage, community health care, involves reciprocal interdependencies that are achieved via integrated management. Scott et al. (2000) also identify medical groups and insurance companies as possible sources of control for integrated systems. While organizational units may be linked (and consolidation and privatization have produced a number of consolidated health care systems), they are not necessarily integrated such that the individual client is able to access different systems of care in order to meet diverse medical and supportive needs.

In contrast to integration, service system fragmentation occurs when there are categorical funding streams that pay for one type of service, but not another, and/or when service agencies focus on only one type of problem or illness (Provan & Sebastian, 1998). Individuals with chronic care conditions need medical and social support services to be integrated because they have multiple needs and are generally unable to navigate an un-integrated service system on their own (Provan & Sebastian, 1998). Community-based coalitions can assist agencies to pool scarce resources and provide a mechanism for joint problem solving (Butterfoss & Kegler, 2012). Another advantage of interorganizational linkages is enhanced opportunities for organizational learning and innovation (Goes & Park, 1997).

Leutz (1999) identifies three levels of integration: linkages, coordination, and full integration. Linkages involve informal sharing and communication about programs, services, and clients between agencies, while coordination involves formalized collaboration that operates informally via partnerships, written agreements, staff cross-training, and shared information systems (Marquart & Konrad, 1996). Full integration can be achieved by either a consolidation of services where some services are centralized within an umbrella organization but agencies retain authority over their services, or via the development of a single authority that operates collectively (Marquart & Konrad,1996). Community-based coalitions involve collaboration and coordination, but stop short of full integration models. Movement from a community coalition to a full integration model would involve some institutionalization and formalization of cooperative arrangements (Butterfoss & Kegler, 2012), which is often difficult, as we will see in this chapter.

In order to determine the level of integration necessary, the client population must be analyzed in terms of the severity, stability, and duration of the illness, the urgency and scope of services required, and clients' ability for self-direction (Leutz, 1999). Informal linkages will work for populations with mild to moderate disabilities; coordination is best suited for those with moderate to severe conditions where care is routine; full integration is necessary for populations with long-term disabilities. Obviously, HIV care necessitates fully integrated systems, but most efforts at integration have been limited to cross-training and the use of multidisciplinary treatment teams. An important exception is the HIV/AIDS Treatment Adherence, Health Outcomes and Cost Study, which I will describe later in the chapter along with other efforts to integrate HIV/AIDS care systems and supports.

The most familiar argument for system integration is Shortell et al. (2000), *Remaking Health Care in America*. A key element of the author's ideal health system is that care is coordinated and integrated across the continuum of care. Systems of care must be holistic in that the "whole" must exist before it can be embedded in each part. Integration will not occur by merely bringing together the parts of the system, rather integration is both a cause and effect of holistic care. Shortell et al. (2000) identifies three mechanisms by which care can be integrated in such a way as to produce holistic systems of care. First is functional integration, which coordinates key support functions (e.g., information systems, financial management, planning, and quality assurance). Second is physician-system integration, where physicians are economically linked to the system and are active participants in planning, management, and governance. There are four types of physician system integration: physician-hospital organizations, management services organizations, medical foundations, and integrated health care organizations (Shortell et al., 2000; Scott et al., 2000). Third is clinical integration where patient care services are coordinated across people, functions, and operating units so as to maximize the value of services delivered. Scott et al., (2000) note that clinical integration involves vertical integration.

However, for care to be coordinated at the provider level (i.e., where the client receives a service), financial and functional integration is necessary. We saw this at the end of Chapter 5: while participants in the cross-training felt they knew how to enhance collaboration with other providers, they felt financial and organizational constraints undermined efforts at collaboration. Clinical care cannot be integrated if organizations are separated by competition for scarce funding, different management structures, different client information systems, and specialization of function. Populations with long-term disabilities and chronic health problems need a number of specialized interventions and coordination among knowledgeable professionals. Clearly, the first obstacle to successful integration is to determine whether the chicken—clinical integration—proceeds or follows the egg—functional integration (Leutz, 1999).

A second major barrier to integration is that efforts to coordinate care are not reimbursable (Anderson & Knickman, 2001). Consequently, managed care represents a major barrier to individual-level integration (i.e., case management, see Chapter 3). At the organizational and systems level, integration must overcome the barriers of vested interests and categorical funding. Furthermore, diverse provider groups must agree on philosophies, as well as standards of care (Cohen, 1998; Vladeck, 2001). Integration is best viewed as a process (rather than an outcome) that involves the sustained commitment of organizations, providers, and fiscal supports.

HIV SYSTEM INTEGRATION

While models of HIV system integration were few and far between prior to the 1990s, the past 10 years has seen a number of reviews and research initiatives. The best known is the HIV/AIDS Treatment Adherence, Health Outcomes and Cost Study (referred to as the HIV Cost Study), which is a federally funded, multi-agency study of integrating HIV, MH, and SA (HIV/AIDS Treatment Adherence, Health Outcomes and Cost Group, 2004). The focus of the HIV Cost Study was to evaluate the efficacy and cost effectiveness of integrated systems of care. Eight research sites, six federal agencies, and one coordinating center collaborated and investigated two primary models of integration: co-location of mental health and substance abuse services with HIV/AIDS medical care, and interagency coordination of care. The specific strategies used at each of the eight research sites and the evaluation instruments are described in an article published in *AIDS Care* (HIV/AIDS Treatment Adherence, Health Outcome and Cost Group, 2004). While not found to be cost effective or to improve patient quality of life (Weaver et al., 2009), the authors do suggest that communities with lower baseline levels of integration than the eight study sites may benefit from integration efforts.

Other researchers have also worked to integrate HIV/AIDS services. An early effort was the Indiana Integration of Care Project (Wright & Shuff, 1995), which was focused on improving integration of the mental health sector with the HIV/AIDS primary care sector. These authors utilize network theory to describe existing levels of integration and the factors that influence integration (i.e., network ties between the two sectors). Rier and Indyk (2006) and Indyk and Rier (2006) describe one inner-city based program that worked to establish interorganizational linkages that bring together agencies, providers, and consumers with different types of expert knowledge in order to improve access to HIV care. Their model, referred to as the geometry of care, has been introduced in other countries and can be modified to work in other communities. More recently, Bauermeister, Tross, and Ehrhardt (2009) have provided a systematic review of system-level efforts to improve HIV prevention and treatment. While most of the studies they reviewed focused on efforts to improve agency infrastructure, several of the studies included collaborative partnerships between agencies. There are also studies of integration efforts in other countries (e.g., Tkatchenko-Schmidt et al., 2010).

In the U.S., the federal government has taken an active role in describing principles and models for integrating systems of care for populations at risk for HIV disease. SAMHSA and its Co-Occurring Center for Excellence (COCE) have provided a series of working papers outlining the principles of system integration. Overview paper 6 (Services Integration) and paper 7 (Systems Integration) are particularly useful and can be easily obtained from SAMHSA (www.coce.samhsa.gov). These working papers summarize existing research and provide a review of major principles for service or system integration. SAMSHA has also provided resources and funding for communities to develop and experiment with different models of integration. In what follows, I describe my experience with one such integration project.

COMMUNITY-BASED EFFORTS TO INTEGRATE HIV, MH, AND SA SERVICES

In October 2000, the Mecklenburg County Public Health Department (located in Charlotte, North Carolina) obtained a planning grant funded from SAMHSA to integrate services to minority populations at risk for HIV disease with co-occurring mental health and substance abuse problems. The planning grant provided $150,000 for 2 years and specifically targeted the active participation of consumers in the planning process. Only six sites in the country were funded; Mecklenburg County was the only single county system to be funded, and also the only urban SMSA.

I was the formative evaluator for the planning grant, and as a sociologist with expertise in organization theory and interorganizational relations, I played a critical role in the development of the integration plan. An Executive Advisory Board (EAB) consisting of representatives of various provider groups and consumers (86 people were on the EAB mailing list) was formed and met monthly to develop a plan. A continuing concern was to bring various minority groups (Black, Hispanic, and Asian) to the table and to elicit active consumer involvement. To this end, an inclusion committee was formed after the first EAB meeting. This committee went out into the community and "brought people to the table." While the majority of the members of the EAB were Black, leaders and consumers from the Hispanic, Asian, and Native American communities were present. There was also diversity in terms of sexual orientation, with consumers and providers who were homosexual and bisexual. There was ongoing concern to reach out into the community and involve individuals who were not accessing services. Early on, it was decided that 50% of the EAB members were to be consumers, a term that included advocates, as well as clients. Grant monies were used to help cover consumer expenses to attend meetings, and to provide reimbursement for time spent working with the EAB. In addition, everyone helped with transportation (I, myself, picked up one consumer for each meeting). Despite these efforts, the majority who regularly attended the EAB meetings (on average, 15 to 20 of the 30 or so attendees) were providers and agency representatives.[1] We constantly worked to increase consumer representation, consumers were clearly present and vocal, and regular attendees to the EAB meetings represented the diversity of background in terms of service needs and minority status.

Meetings were participatory and early efforts to define a common vision (and, ultimately, a mission statement) and objectives for attaining that vision were led by a facilitator who ensured the active involvement of everyone at each stage of the planning. Early in the planning process, we held a workshop to develop a mission statement, and this workshop achieved the ideal goal of 50% consumer participation (as did later efforts to refine the mission statement at community forums). Each of the 40 EAB members attending the workshop was asked to write down the key elements of a mission, their vision, and their beliefs about the EAB. A list of common beliefs was identified, and then individuals were placed into three groups to develop their own mission statements (groups included equal mixes of providers or agency staff, consumers, and advocates). All three statements were placed on large poster paper, and considered at length. The best one was selected by a majority vote, and then another hour was spent making modifications. At each meeting, the mission statement was read, and time was given for any modifications (several occurred early on). The final project mission is as follows:

> Consumers and professionals will work collaboratively to provide an integrated system of prevention and treatment that will address the interrelated needs of persons facing the challenges of HIV/AIDS, substance abuse, and mental illness.

Following the development of the mission statement, the EAB clarified its role and responsibilities, and ways that decisions based on consensus would be made. There were several discussions that illustrated "turf" battles (i.e., domain disputes). For example, key agencies asked how the EAB was different than the Regional HIV/AIDS Consortium, or from the health department. It was agreed that the EAB would work to develop an integration plan, foster consumer involvement, identify underserved populations, recognize other partners and keep them informed, provide a bridge between agencies and other initiatives, and help break down "turf."

Before developing an integration plan, the EAB had to map existing services and identify gaps in services. Furthermore, there was a need to synthesize existing data and reports in order to identify what information needed to be collected (this was primarily my responsibility). While data was being collected and assessed, the EAB defined the key elements of an integration plan: prevention, integration, cross-training, and cross-cultural access. Subcommittees were developed (each representative of specific populations and service sectors), and work began on an integration plan that addressed each of these four areas. I attended all subcommittee meetings and worked to integrate various elements of the developing integration plan. The process of collecting data and developing a preliminary plan took most of spring 2001, during which the EAB also was planning a community forum. A community forum was one of the features specified in the grant as a means to elicit community participation in the planning process.

The community forum was held in a church in a largely minority neighborhood with high rates of HIV/AIDS. The forum began with breakfast, provided lunch, and ended at 4:30 p.m. There were 47 participants who attended the morning session and worked in breakout groups. Only ten of these participants were EAB members, so the goal of obtaining increased community involvement was successful. Participation dwindled after lunch, although there were still over 32 participants in the afternoon sessions who completed an evaluation instrument from which we know the majority of the participants were providers (81%), and the majority of these providers represented HIV agencies (56.3%). The majority (62%) of the respondents were Black, and there were representatives of the Hispanic, Asian, and Native American communities.

Rather than merely present the preliminary integration plan, the same facilitator who assisted with the development of a mission statement led the group in the development of its own plan to increase collaboration. The four priority areas (prevention, cross-cultural competence, cross-training, and integration) were identified, and participants self-selected into one of these groups for the morning session. A facilitator was assigned to each group to keep track of the ideas developed and to present that group's consensus on gaps in the system and barriers to collaboration to the larger group before lunch. The groups ranged from 16 members (prevention) to 8 members (integration). In the afternoon, the groups met again to develop specific strategies to improve the system in terms of their priority area. There was a great deal of overlap with ideas that had been generated and shared at EAB meetings, and the results of the forum were integrated with the preliminary integration plan.

Following the forum, task groups consisting of consumers and providers were formed around each aspect of the integration plan. These task groups met weekly through the summer to work out the details of the integration plan and to apply for the SAMSHA implementation funding. Other sources of funding were also explored. I was a member of all of the task groups, and brought my understanding of system integration, as well as barriers to such integration, to the table. I helped the group to determine current levels of system integration, and to determine what level of integration was ideal and what was feasible. The final integration plan is presented in Appendix C. The plan specifies an overall objective of treating and educating as many HIV/SA/MH clients and potential clients as quickly as possible through a client-centered holistic approach, and how the current system of cooperation (the existing level of integration) would move toward a more fully integrated state with an interagency coordinating body; multidisciplinary, multi-agency case management teams; cross-training of providers and consumers; culturally appropriate and sensitive materials; and an emphasis on prevention and outreach to minority populations at risk for HIV disease.

In terms of the level of integration desired, consumers actively sought the one-stop shop model, where all of their health care needs could be met at one place. Providers found this system of care idealistic, and were also opposed to various types of consolidation where there was some centralization of authority. This opposition had two sources: conflict between the two obvious choices for an umbrella organization, and concern that organizational specialization and inefficiencies of either umbrella organization would be replicated. The model agreed on by both providers and consumers was that of "no wrong door," in that whatever agency a consumer might turn to, they would be able to obtain the full array of services needed. Consequently, the integration plan reflects a more practical orientation toward coordination (rather than full integration), which would be achieved by the development of a coordinator position; an interagency, multidisciplinary treatment team; professional cross-training; and common standards of care.

However, SAMHSA was not able to provide implementation monies (due to a change of political environment) and the integration plan was not funded. Consequently, formal mechanisms for integration were not put into place. Nor were the members of the EAB able to arrive at consensus for local efforts to achieve integration beyond continued cross-training. Without additional funding, key agencies were not supportive of the multi-agency, multidisciplinary treatment team, as they did not want to give up ownership of their clients, nor could they afford to let key staff take time to work on an interagency treatment team. Stakeholders also feared a coordinator position would simply add on another layer of bureaucracy, and raised questions about where such a position would be housed. Without additional funding, agencies could not take on any more work, although it is obvious that the existence of the EAB and the time spent planning had indeed improved system-level coordination in a number of ways.

CONTINUED COMMUNITY-BASED EFFORTS TO INTEGRATE SYSTEMS OF CARE: THE HIV TASK FORCE

After the grant ended, the EAB continued to meet and it was decided this body should be a consumer-run advisory board. However, consumers did not step up to the table, and the board came to an end. Providers continued to meet in a variety of ways, and in fall 2003, an HIV Task Force was developed with the support of the health department, which is under the authority of the Mecklenburg County Commissioners. The charge given to the Task Force was to develop a set of recommendations for a "broad based, comprehensive community plan to eliminate HIV disease in Mecklenburg County" (Mecklenburg County HIV Task Force, 2004). The Task Force was to operate under guidelines developed by the Centers for Disease Control for community prevention planning, and the strategic plan was to be in accordance with state and federal guidelines and planning efforts, and reflect consultation and input from HIV and community health advocates and stakeholders.

There was a great deal of effort to involve consumers, as well as all members of the community. The ground rules established at the first meeting were:

1. Your Voice Counts
2. Dialogue, not Debate
3. Respect Time
4. Let's Get Started
5. No Interruptions
6. All are HIV Equal

We had several meetings that can be described as little more than collective catharsis in which grievances and complaints were aired. People took full advantage of the rules, "Your Voice Counts" and "No Interruptions," which was an ongoing source of frustration to me as it violated the "Respect Time" rule. Meetings were attended by 20 to 30 individuals, and membership was not consistent, so there was a need to continually rehash old issues and listen to new voices. However, we did acquire an audience before the Health and Safety subcommittee of the County Commissioners, and consequently had to prepare a formal presentation. I was asked to lead the first community-based meeting to prepare the presentation and was able to put the many ideas generated in previous brainstorming sessions into an outline (using a large poster-board and newsprint). When we moved to formalize the presentation, participation dwindled to a few agency heads, the health department epidemiologist, and myself. Over several more meetings, we prepared a presentation that documented the growing problem of HIV disease in the county, and the many gaps in services. The director of the health department also developed a policy statement that ultimately asked the County Commissioners to "acknowledge the seriousness of the HIV disease epidemic" and to provide leadership in the development of a plan to address this problem.

Community advocates joined us for the public presentation, which stretched to three meetings due to the many interruptions from the more conservative members of the county subcommittee. A couple of shouting matches ensued, which were entertaining to say the least. Advocates were enraged by what they perceived as the ignorance and racism of some of the County Commissioners, and seemed to feel that somehow they could be "educated." We were ultimately granted an audience in front of the entire Board of County Commissioners (these meetings are held at night and are televised), and in addition to the consumers who had presented their stories to the Health and Safety subcommittee, we had esteemed members of the medical community who attested to the threat the community faced if some action were not taken to reduce the growth of HIV disease in the county. The presentation was a success in that we were granted authority to develop a plan to "eliminate HIV disease in Mecklenburg County," and were provided with as many lunches and snacks as needed to achieve our goal.

The strategic plan was to address three areas: prevention, care, and the system of delivery. Three subcommittees were formed around each area, and I was selected to be chair of the System of Delivery subcommittee. The HIV Task Force spent a great deal of time preparing a strategic plan on HIV disease in Mecklenburg County that was presented to the County Commissioners in an ongoing effort to confront the problems posed by HIV and the inability of the existing service system to deal with the growing need for integrated systems. The health department played a major role in providing the Task Force with specific guidelines and in preparing the final report, which provided a thorough analysis of the epidemiology of HIV disease and its impact in Mecklenburg County. The key components of the integration plan were evident in the strategic plan: integrated service delivery with mental health and substance abuse, enhancement of existing levels of collaboration among providers, linguistic and cultural competency, and an emphasis on prevention and outreach.

The System of Delivery plan first reviewed existing data on systems of care. This data was organized and presented in a manner so as to be user-friendly and easy to read. Next, we reviewed best practices for integrating health care systems. Mecklenburg County is unique in that it was the site for two major demonstration projects for system integration: the Robert Wood Johnson Foundation Program for Chronic Mental Illness (1985–1992) and the ACCESS Project for Homeless Populations (1991–1996). This summary of data highlighted the existence of system fragmentation, and identified mechanisms of system integration (described previously). We then provided a list of very specific recommendations that had been agreed on by the entire HIV Task Force.

The first thing we asked for was the formation of an HIV Community Council that would bring together consumers, providers, advocates, decision makers and policy leaders to ensure that the system of delivery was meeting the needs of those individuals whose lives are affected by HIV disease. The more general goal for system integration was a "coordinated and appropriately funded system of service delivery that optimizes resources and prevents missed opportunities for testing, counseling, treatment, and service referral" (Mecklenburg County HIV Task Force, 2004, p. 10). Specifically, the Task Force asked for cross-training of providers in HIV, mental health, and substance abuse; early intervention counseling; and expanded referral to HIV providers. In addition, attention had to be given to the provision of culturally appropriate care and outreach to high-risk minority communities. We identified those resources that would be needed to redress existing system fragmentations: funding for a service coordinator, development of a common client information system, the development of client assessment tools, and financial support for interagency cross-training.

The Task Force did get additional resources for the health department based on their recommendations (i.e., more money for outreach and testing in minority communities and six new case manager positions). The County Commissioners approved our request for an HIV Council and charged the HIV Council to develop specific strategies and recommendations for a broad-based comprehensive plan for prevention, care, and system integration. Council membership follows the guidelines for advisory boards outlined by the Centers for Disease Control. More specifically, Council membership consists of 20 to 25 members who represent those most heavily impacted by HIV/AIDS, as well as the professional HIV/AIDS community. Members are elected and serve 3-year terms. The Council bylaws and first board were approved in summer 2006, and the Council has been active since with bimonthly meetings and several public events each year (e.g., an HIV/AIDS Health Fair, and several community forums). The HIV Council has also reported before the County Commissioners on a regular basis to provide them with updated information about the prevalence and impact of

HIV disease in the county. I have served as secretary of the Council since its formation in 2006. However, there has been little progress toward improving system integration.

CONCLUSION AND DISCUSSION: COMMUNITY-BASED COALITIONS AND SYSTEM INTEGRATION

Despite over 10 years of intensive planning (2000 to 2013), formal mechanisms for integration have not been put into place, largely because of the lack of funding for specific mechanisms needed to integrate diverse systems. Even had funding been available, there were key debates over who would have controlled these funds, and hence, who would control the process of integration. These debates point to the limitations of the coalitions developed to pursue system-level integration. In terms of the Integration plan, while many assumed the health department was the logical place to house the coordinator position, as well as the multi-agency, multidisciplinary team, other agencies and many consumers were wary of the bureaucratic policies of the health department. Furthermore, providers were not willing to hand their clients over to a coordinator that did not operate within their agency or to another case management team. In short, while grass roots consensus was reached at a variety of levels, issues of governance and authority for system integration, as identified by Marquarat and Konrad (1996), were not resolved. This failure was due to pre-existing domain disputes that were not resolved, largely because these disputes arise from functional specialization between providers that are maintained by inadequate categorical funding streams. Limited resources and inadequate funding were early recognized as key problems, for which no easy solution exists.

Ultimately, neither the Integration EAB nor the HIV Task Force were fully able to resolve the domain disputes that would have enabled true system-wide reform. Drawing from the model developed by Butterfoss and Kegler (2012) for coalitions, the EAB never moved beyond the first stage of formation and member engagement; although the Task Force did move to the second stage of maintenance by having the County Commissioners recognize and support an HIV Council. It remains to be seen if the HIV Council can move to full institutionalization and sustainability. Shortell et al. (2002) identify the key components of successful community partnerships in their evaluation of 25 programs in the Community Care Network Demonstration Project. These projects were all designed to improve community health; and central to successful programs is both an explicit vision of what can be accomplished, as well as a structure that recognizes the complexities of maintaining interorganizational ties over time.

In the cross-training described in Chapter 5, participants identified the key components of a collaborative network: commitment, representation, and agreement on goals and roles. All of these factors existed following both periods of planning for HIV system integration. However, participants also identified challenges to collaborative networks for each of these three components (see Chapter 5). While planning groups may be committed, there are always unresolved conflicts, existing hierarchies, and domain disputes that need to be openly acknowledged and resolved before community planning can proceed. In terms of representation, debates over who makes decisions and levels of authority, or hierarchy, also reflect ongoing power differences. Agreement on goals and roles are also limited by participants emphasizing their needs, and, once again, domain disputes between agencies and participants. As noted by one EAB member in the final evaluation, there is "naiveté about hidden agendas" among providers. In both planning efforts described above, the health department had the power and controlled scarce resources for planning efforts, and while planning was inclusive, there was still a great deal of distrust of the health department, which was generally seen as "big brother." The professional culture of an organized bureaucracy can undermine demands for equity and participatory decision-making. Full institutionalization of community-based coalitions requires strong leadership and staffing for long-term sustainability (Butterfoss & Kegler, 2012). Disputes over who can provide that leadership will certainly undercut efforts for system integration. Shortell et al. (2002) describe a three-component leadership structure. First, there is a committed core leader or leaders who can articulate a shared vision and earn the respect of the coalition members. Second is a consistent organization driver, generally an organization such as the health department, which can provide continuity over time. Third, successful programs were able to delegate specific tasks or specific problems to subsidiary leaders or groups. There also needs to be clear rules and procedures for dealing with conflict, and a clear statement and understanding of each participant's vested interests. Finally, there also needs to be a communication plan that allows individuals a voice in the collaborative process. As Shortell et al. (2002) emphasize, it takes ongoing organizational efforts to manage size, diversity, and conflict for coalitions to be able to succeed in accomplishing their goals.

Returning to community efforts in Mecklenburg County, while formal mechanisms to integrate HIV systems of care were not implemented, there is no doubt that working toward the goal of integration is good for the system. The true measure of system integration is providers who recognize, and work to overcome, turf battles. Does the HIV provider know who to call for a mental health referral, or for substance abuse treatment? Is the mental health provider comfortable discussing HIV disease, and does this person know where to send a client for testing? Does the infectious disease clinic know how to assess for mental illness, so that they do not prescribe medications that may interact with medications for schizophrenia or depression? Can the substance abuse provider overcome professional biases against harm reduction models, and work with HIV providers to get their clients on HIV medication and treatment?

Health system integration and community-based coalition building should be thought of as a process (Hassett & Austin, 1997). Interagency teams and coordinating councils have been found to foster greater interorganizational exchanges (Foster-Fishman, Salem, Allen, & Fahrbach, 2001), and community-based programs lead to stronger interorganizational relationships (McGuire, Rosenheck, & Burnette, 2002). Continued engagement to achieve common purposes can potentially overcome domain disputes and open the door for more systematic efforts to integrate the diverse services needed by minority populations at risk for HIV disease. Any type of attempt to integrate services brings people to the table, where information and ideas can be exchanged, and it is this exchange of information that is the core element of an integrated system.

However, managed care also works against system integration and makes it harder, if not impossible, for providers to work effectively together. As seen with the HIV Cost Study, an emphasis on clinical efficacy and cost effectiveness (both key features of managed care) does not necessarily coincide with the goals of system integration and improved client outcomes, which are not easily measured. The only way a managed care system can attain integration is with some form of centralized authority that manages the entire pool of resources for the diverse services needed by chronic care populations. Otherwise, categorical funding streams, different eligibility criteria, and diverse client information systems work against any form of clinical integration. More fundamentally, managed care is based on a medical model with a focus on short-term treatment for acute conditions, or else crises intervention. The future of the health care system is uncertain, and time will tell if managed care can meet the challenges of chronic illness and long-term care.

NOTE

1. Meetings were held at 9 a.m. in the health department in the first year of the grant, and this was certainly a barrier for many EAB members. However, it was critical to have agency representation as we sought pathways to greater system collaboration. In the second year of the grant, we moved meetings to the afternoon at a center for HIV and SA services, and consumer participation increased markedly. This fit with the natural flow of the planning process as we moved from planning to seeking strategies to implement our general integration strategies.

7 Advancing Advocacy
Moving from the Client to the System

WORLD AIDS DAY

World AIDS Day was finally acknowledged in Charlotte in 2010. The HIV Council described in the previous chapter had worked all fall to plan a public display and reading of an HIV Proclamation by the County Commissioners. It took a lot of effort to make something happen on World AIDS Day. First, we presented an update and report on HIV disease to the Health and Community Safety Committee of the County Commissioners in May 2010. This was followed by a public presentation to the entire Board of County Commissioners in September. We worked hard on a presentation that combined factual information with firsthand accounts, and asked for the County Commissioners to read a public proclamation in support of efforts to reduce new incidence of HIV/AIDS, and to have a public display to raise awareness of the impact of HIV disease in the community on World AIDS Day. The presentation was extremely well received by insiders, the public, and the County Commissioners. Our requests were granted—we were "on" for World AIDS Day. The public display would be of shoes, with each pair of shoes representing a new HIV case in 2010. Termed "Sole 2 Soul," the public display of shoes had been present at each of the 2010 HIV/AIDS Awareness Days and was the result of grassroots community organizing, with some support from the HIV Council. The shoes would be displayed at the Government Center, and one of the County Commissioners would read the Proclamation (see Appendix D) after a four-block public march from the center of downtown to the Government Center.

Traditionally, the Regional AIDS Interfaith Network (RAIN) had commemorated World AIDS Day with a public reading of names of those who had died in the past year. We decided to move beyond "remembrance" to "resilience" as the new theme for World AIDS Day, just as HIV disease has moved from a largely fatal disease to a long-term chronic disease. Resilience means to survive from illness. We started at the traditional downtown site for the reading of the names with a wreath of "remembrance" and a brief invocation. Those gathered (about 30 individuals) then carried the wreath and a number of banners and signs four city blocks to the Government

Center. There awaited the display of shoes, the wreath of "resilience," and more posters and information.

It was cold and windy, but sunny. The wreaths and posters kept falling down, but we all huddled together and listened to a number of exceptional speakers. Nothing had been planned except some words about testing from a representative from the health department and the reading of the Proclamation. However, individuals stepped up—with song, with prayer, with thanks, with anger, with passion. The display of shoes had the desired effect; the diversity of shoes represented certainly gave a visual message about the impact of HIV disease in the community. Informational posters provided the details and facts. In closing, an invocation of resilience was read. We were moved, silent, then hugging each other. Despite the cold and wind, people lingered. It was a success.

FROM HIV CARE PROVIDERS TO ADVOCATES

In January 2011, the Executive Committee of the HIV Council met to plan events for the coming year. Yes, World AIDS Day was a success. Yes, the display of shoes was a success and furthered testing and educational goals. Yes, the County Commissioners had listened to us. But funding was even scarcer. Most Ryan White dollars had been diverted to agencies able to provide medical care, away from the traditional community-based organizations that had provided supportive services for so many years. Ryan White monies were to be used in a very clearly defined manner to support primarily medical care (rather than the social support services deemed so necessary for comprehensive HIV care). Changes in Medicaid rules would further limit the ability of these agencies to support case management services (see Chapter 3). Could we continue to do outreach and encourage testing if there were no services? After an hour of discussion, the members of the Executive Committee became passionate; first angry, then frustrated, but then angry again. It was time to move beyond planning to advocacy—we had to do more.

Let me step back from the Council to a more analytical level. As I revise and update this book, we are slowly recovering from a severe recession. Joblessness is still high, and public revenue is severely limited at all levels. With higher levels of unemployment, there is more poverty and more unmeet need. It has been a very rough couple of years for all kinds of CBOs and service providers. With funding restrictions, service providers have been struggling to stay afloat, trying to maintain some level of care for clients, and to obtain money for outreach and education. I conducted a Needs Assessment for the Ryan White Transitional Grant Area in summer 2013, and the results point to growing gaps in services. We interviewed representatives from 20 HIV agencies (half received Ryan White funding and the other half did not). Over half of the agencies (60%) reported a net loss in funding in the past year, and 50% of the respondents felt the system of services had gotten worse in the past 2 years. In an open-ended question about specific reasons for the decline in the HIV system of care, almost everyone mentioned a decline in funding as the primary reason. Furthermore, 57% of the respondents did not think there was adequate access to HIV care, and 56% also felt access was worse than it was 2 years ago.

It does not look as though public funding will be restored any time soon, so maybe it is time to move beyond maintaining the status quo to efforts to change the entire system. Rather than incremental piecemeal approaches, perhaps we need something that is more comprehensive. As articulated by one agency representative interviewed for the Needs Assessment, "policy and funding are focused on short-term solutions . . . rather than focusing on the long-term costs of inadequate care." Rather than advocating for their clients, providers may need to engage in more broad-based political action that is directed toward changing the system.

Historically, HIV/AIDS care had been the result of a great deal of advocacy on the part of patients (Epstein, 1996). Lune (2007) provides an excellent account of HIV/AIDS and community organizing in New York City. He notes that HIV/AIDS brought together a "wide assortment of socially marginalized groups," which mobilized and developed community-based organizations that developed models of care (Lune, 2007, p. 4). As has been so well documented, federal and local governments were originally not at all interested in HIV/AIDS care. One result of early advocacy efforts was the Ryan White CARE Act of 1990, which brought federal dollars to HIV care providers. However, it brought greater governmental control of these services. Lune (2007) does an excellent job telling the story of the conflict between the state and the community; between public and private responses to HIV disease. Providers receiving federal and state dollars are prevented from outright public advocacy, and have focused their efforts on obtaining grants and funding to support their services. While individual agencies receiving public dollars for services may not be able to engage in advocacy, consumers can and they have. AIDS advocacy is widely recognized as one of the more successful patient advocacy efforts (Hoffman, Tomes, Grob, & Schlesinger, 2011). But today, many HIV/AIDS consumers are largely disenfranchised, and fight daily to maintain their health and well being.[1] As noted by Hoffman et al. (2011, p. 13), patient empowerment takes place in an environment of "pervasive social and economic inequality. Differences of power, income, resources, and access to the media shape the ability of patient groups to affect policy."

We can't look to a widespread consumer-led movement to address the challenges of a fragmented health care system; instead, we need broad-based coalitions of consumers, advocates, and providers. While individual agencies and community-based organizations may not engage in direct advocacy on behalf of their clients because of their reliance on public funding, interorganizational groups (such as the HIV Council) can engage in advocacy. Furthermore, broad-based coalitions are also in the position to say something about the entire system of care—not just the needs of individual consumers or agencies. It is too early to say, but hopefully, World AIDS Day 2010 sparked a flame that will spread. However, advocacy work is difficult, and in the following section, I move to a discussion of the conflicts faced by researchers who work with community groups to improve social structures and reduce health inequities—the focus of most community-based participatory action research.

THE ROLE OF THE RESEARCHER IN COMMUNITY-BASED PARTICIPATORY ACTION RESEARCH

A major question for the participatory action researcher is what role they are to play in the community. Specifically, the community-based action researcher faces the dilemmas posed by assuming either a "priestly" or a "prophetic" role. As first defined by Friedrichs (1970), "priests" adhere to scientific canon and collect data on how the social world operates in a value-neutral manner. "Prophets" seek to change the world, and use theory and research to affect social reforms. As an academic sociologist, my work has largely been of the "priestly" variety, although relevant to social policy. For example, some of my past work on the response of businesses to the Americans with Disabilities Act was presented to Equal Employment Opportunity Commission chair, Paul Miller. While I have been asked at times to assume a prophetic role, I have remained pretty firmly in the priestly role and try to provide the community with the data and frameworks they need to affect reforms to the system.

Community groups also face the conflicts posed by a priestly versus a prophetic role. In terms of their approaches to social change, I have observed an interesting difference between providers and consumers. Providers tend to be "priests"—seeking only to work within the confines of the existing system; consumers are generally "prophets"—seeking major reforms and system-wide changes. During the integration project, consumers actively sought the one-stop shop model where all of their health care needs could be met at one place. This is the model of system integration advocated by the U.S. Department of Health and Human Services (Center for Substance Abuse Treatment, 2007). Providers found this system of care idealistic, and were also opposed to various types of consolidation where there was some centralization of authority. The model agreed on by both providers and consumers was that of "no wrong door," in that whatever agency a consumer might turn to, they would be able to obtain the full array of services needed. Consequently, the integration plan described in Chapter 6 reflects a more practical orientation toward collaboration that would be achieved by the development of a coordinator position; an interagency, multidisciplinary treatment team; professional cross-training; and common standards of care.

Within the HIV Task Force, conflicts between priests and prophets were even more apparent. The Chair of the Task Force was a physician, and clearly of the "priestly" data-driven species. The Associate Chair was a well-known community advocate and religious leader, although trained at the CDC and possessing a Ph.D. While she was "priestly" in her orientation to scientifically validated interventions, she played the role of the "prophet" on the Task Force and was seen as a community leader advocating for social change. Besides the usual kinds of turf battles I had encountered in the integration project, there was ongoing conflict over how best to make a case to the County Commissioners. Many advocates wanted to make their appeals on a personal, emotional level. They were disdainful of previous research or reports, or any kind of authority beyond that of lived experience. The more pragmatic (myself included) felt the only way to convince the County Commissioners to confront the problems of HIV disease (and, ultimately, give us some much-needed resources) was to make a factual case based on existing data and economic forecasts. Our presentations ultimately combined both forms of insight and data.

A second source of conflict was whether to ask for major system reform (including restructuring the role of the County Commissioners as the Board of Health) or whether to ask for resources to make incremental changes to the system. In short, there was further conflict between the prophets and the priests. We had numerous meetings of each of the subgroups and the larger Task Force, where the same issues were raised again and again. There was also conflict over the framing of the issues and the language used in the plan. Just to give one example, people argued about whether to use the term culturally sensitive, culturally relevant, culturally competent, or culturally effective. Similar arguments arose about the use of the term minority. The debates became more heated when targeting specific programs (needle exchange, sex education in the schools, HIV testing in jails). These same debates had also characterized the development of the integration plan. Had I embarked on my advocacy role as a prophet, I feel I would have been sorely disappointed with the result. As a priest, I could cheer when we voted to approve our plan, and be able to maintain the needed objectivity and distance to help negotiate a consensus and present a unified front to the County Commissioners.

Many sociology departments have dispute resolution as part of their applied sociology programs, and there is literature on sociologists developing mediation techniques in order to serve as community facilitators (Capece & Schantz, 2000). I found that the skills described by Capece and Schantz (2000) were indeed critical to my advocacy role. First, there is a need to de-emphasize your role as an expert.[2] I had initially approached my advocacy role as a "priest," feeling my contribution would be to provide social facts. I gathered needed data, drafted multiple reports, tried to organize ideas and opinions, rarely got on the podium myself, and never offered my own opinion. But I learned to put aside my priestly belief that facts can speak for themselves, and to acknowledge that in the political arena, people's values let them ignore or distort the facts. Even when the facts supported the advocates' position, they wanted a message that would be "felt," not merely heard. My research skills were not as valuable as my ability to help individuals negotiate consensus—to learn to agree to disagree and present a unified voice.

Capece and Schantz (2000) argue that the second essential skill a mediator must have is the ability to separate individuals from their emotions and positions, and to reframe issues in terms of larger community needs. This distance is essential to negotiated consensus, and was particularly difficult for the prophets. The priests among the group worked hard to negotiate agreement among diverse groups and individuals, and to help them present their ideas in a format that would reflect this consensus and to also make a pervasive case for reform. However, this consensus was fragile. Even when a professional facilitator helped the community to develop a mission and a plan to achieve this mission that apparently had a great deal of consensus, the consensus disappeared without any external pressure to present a unified voice. As noted by Strauss (1978), consensus needs to be continually reconstituted. However, this continual renegotiation contributes to a sense of frustration that goes beyond aggravation and can lead to a sense of futility. I am not sure that I have made a difference in the local community and its efforts to address the many problems posed by HIV/AIDS. It is too soon to tell if the County Commissioners will make any changes, but we will continue to advocate and I can only hope that these efforts will open the door to larger system-wide reforms.

UNDERSTANDING THE IDEOLOGICAL ROOTS OF SYSTEM FRAGMENTATION

Service system fragmentation occurs when there are categorical funding streams that pay for one type of service, but not another, and/or when service agencies focus on only one type of problem or illness (Provan & Sebastian, 1998). Obviously, one reason agencies only focus on one type of illness is because that reflects their area of expertise, as well as their primary funding source. Expertise and funding are obviously linked. Both sources of system fragmentation originate in categorical thinking about diseases, which divides heath care providers even more fundamentally than professional boundaries, and has also driven different funding allocations for each illness or social need. A core question facing HIV providers and leaders is whether Ryan White funding for HIV care will ultimately be rolled into Medicaid streams with the implementation of the Affordable Care Act. This is not likely in the near future (given that so many states have not accepted Medicaid expansion), but is a distinct possibility in the future. Most providers feel HIV care needs separate funding (and more of it), but this certainly adds to overall system fragmentation, as most HIV clients need comprehensive physical and behavioral health care—not just HIV care.

As articulated by Rosenberg (2007), our current view of disease is based on the use of disease categories, whereby diagnosis is linked to disease specificity. That is, diseases are discrete entities, reflecting objective categories that reside outside the experience of illness. Mishler (1989) provides a concise summary of the central propositions that constitute the disease (or biomedical) model:

1. A biological definition of disease: A disease is accounted for by deviations from a biological norm.
2. The doctrine of specific etiology: Diseases can be ordered into a taxonomy based on symptoms, symptoms can be clustered into syndromes, and syndromes into diseases with specific pathologies.
3. The assumption of generic disease: Each disease has unique and distinguishing features that are universally recognized.
4. The scientific neutrality of medicine: Decisions about diagnosis are neutral and based on standards of objectivity and rationality.

Rosenberg (2007) does an excellent job of unpacking assumptions 1 through 3, and explicitly focuses on chronic care conditions where the doctrine of disease specificity is "especially problematic" (p. 30). In particular, he notes that AIDS elucidates "the arbitrariness of conventional distinctions between the cultural and biological, the disciplinary boundaries historically separating sociology, ecology, and biology" (pp. 154–155). Rosenberg (2007) advocates a new type of holism, which prioritizes a multidimensional view of the patient as a person (not a disease). This argument is not new; leading medical sociologists have argued for some time that the disease model is not appropriate for the care of chronic illness (Kleinman, 1988; Mechanic, 1995; Strauss et al., 1985). However, we have yet to develop an alternative theoretical framework.

Freidson (1984) addresses the fourth postulate identified by Mishler, and focuses on medicine as a social institution—a moral enterprise—that is dominated by professionals who seek to maintain professional autonomy and control (and, thereby, status and prestige, as well as income). Abbott (1988) has extended Freidson's work to provide a stronger framework for understanding jurisdictional disputes and professional boundaries. Clearly, domain disputes are important to understanding system fragmentation, as well as failures to integration efforts, especially clinical integration (see Chapter 6 for a description of diverse forms of integration). Clinical integration is critical to chronic care populations (Shortell et al., 2000), and emerges where patient care services are integrated across people, functions, and organizations in such a way that the values of services delivered is maximized. Another way of describing clinical integration is a patient-centered, or holistic, system of care. However, diverse provider groups must agree on philosophies of care, as well as standards of care, and while providers may agree on the language of holistic care, much more work is needed for them to overcome disciplinary and organization boundaries that prioritize disease specificity, which is then reinforced by jurisdictional disputes. As described by Timmermans and Berg (2003, p. 203):

> Work around patient trajectories is fragmented because of intra and inter-organizational borders that have much relation with organizations' and professions' histories, but little with the needs of individual patients. . . . Tasks are not aligned; organizational routines do not articulate with one another; information is not shared.

As so well described by people I have worked with in provider cross-training, "Our approaches to patient care are an inch wide and a mile deep." This is seen as a major barrier to holistic patient care by providers. However, providers also need to move beyond holistic care at the client level to "wholistic" care at the systems level.[3]

Clinical integration (holistic care) necessitates functional integration (wholistic care), which emerges where key support services are coordinated across all of the operating organizations in a system of care (Shortell et al., 2000). Key support services include financial management, information systems, and planning. In other words, clinical care cannot be integrated if organizations are separated by competition for scarce funding, different management structures, different client information systems, and specialization of function or task. Nor can patient advocacy advance the claims of diverse patient groups that do not share a common identity (Hoffman et al., 2011). Rather than professional boundaries, funding is a key barrier to functional coordination—that is why cross-training cannot achieve system integration. In addition, efforts to coordinate patient care are generally not reimbursable (Anderson & Knickman, 2001), and managed care has certainly increased system fragmentation, as the primary incentive for any managed care mechanism is to shift costs. Coming full circle, managed care is also based on a biomedical model that not only prioritizes disease specificity, but also focuses on short-term, efficacious treatments—even for chronic care populations (Schlesinger & Mechanic, 1993).

By reinforcing treatment for only those health conditions for which there is a medical diagnosis, and treatment is medically efficacious, managed care reinforces the process of medicalization. Increasingly, "managed care organizations are an arbiter of what is deemed medically appropriate or inappropriate" (Conrad, 2007, p. 141), although Conrad notes that managed care has also placed constraints on medicalization by limiting some treatments that are not medically efficacious. Medicalization reinforces categorical approaches to health care, funding specific treatments for specific diseases, and increasing system fragmentation. Medicalization is also dominant in our human services system—only services that deal with medical problems are paid for (Conrad, 2007). This is strikingly evident in the recent restrictions on Ryan White dollars—three-quarters of Ryan White dollars must be used for those services (even case management) clearly defined as meeting medical objectives.

Medicalization has merged with market forces, especially pharmaceutical firms (Conrad, 2007). Increasingly, diseases (such as anxiety) are marketed in order to sell profitable medications. I am sure every HIV/AIDS patient is indeed anxious, but medication is probably not the best solution to the very real sources of their anxiety. In this marketing of disease, pharmaceutical firms have been able to change the biological standards for "normal," thereby increasing the number of those who deviate from the norm (e.g., witness new hypertension and cholesterol guidelines). Perhaps more critically, medical and health services research also reflect medicalization trends—the solution to HIV or mental illness lies not in changes to social systems or better systems of prevention and treatment, but in new medications that provide a biological cure. Consequently, medicalization provides a mediatory myth (mediatory myths help bridge contradictions), whereby research and funding is believed to be directed toward cure, giving both providers and patients hope, but not fundamentally challenging domain assumptions that work against wholistic care. The dominance of objective disease categories (and cures) obscures the "conflicted relationships among medicine's moral, technical, and market identities" (Rosenberg, 2007, p. 31).

A THEORETICAL FRAMEWORK FOR WHOLISTIC CARE

I return to current conceptions about comprehensive care (co-morbidity and cumulative disadvantage) introduced in Chapter 1, which provide frameworks for understanding the multiple needs of individual clients, but do not really provide models for wholistic care. Closely related to both co-morbidity and cumulative disadvantage is the theoretical framework of intersectionality. Intersectionality begins with the reality of multiple identities, and focuses on how gender, race, social class and other social statuses and identities intersect (Bowleg, 2012). As such, intersectionality has a clear affinity with the more medical concept of co-morbidity, where various illnesses intersect, and is also focused primarily on the individual level. However, Bowleg (2012) argues that intersectionality focuses on oppressed groups, and hence allows for an understanding of how systems of inequality at the macro level impact individual experiences and identities, although there is no theoretical guidance on how to link these two levels. While an important theoretical perspective for public health (Bowleg, 2012), not much research has moved beyond the micro level of multiple intersecting social statuses. Specific to HIV, Wyatt et al. (2013) develop an intersectional model of gender, race, and HIV risk and resilience (p. 250) that provides some guidance for HIV researchers. I agree that the framework of intersectionality is critical, especially for understanding the source of health disparities, but there needs to be a general framework to understand how social structures indeed intersect with individual identities, and I have some suggestions for how to think about this in what follows.

I suggest a framework for system integration and health reform that builds on earlier systems models as developed by Talcott Parsons (1960). In particular, I use his framework for examining the interplay of culture, society, and the individual. This model is depicted in Figure 7.1, and I suggest it is a useful framework for addressing the kind of healthcare reforms that will indeed result in wholistic systems of care. At the cultural level, we have beliefs that legitimatize ideological assumptions about the disease model and medicalization, as well as those that reinforce stigma. At the societal level, we have rationalized bureaucratic structures that are organized around profit-based motives. At the societal level, we also have conditions of poverty and inadequate access to health care. At the individual level are individuals living with HIV (or any other patient population living with a chronic care condition), and understanding of the stress processes and social supports is critical to improving their quality of life.

This model also provides an organizing framework for empirical research. Rather than merely focus on patient outcomes or health disparities, researchers can map the complex ways that ideological beliefs, stigma, health care, social supports, and patient outcomes are interrelated. This model can also be used to think about how the micro (the individual patient), meso (the

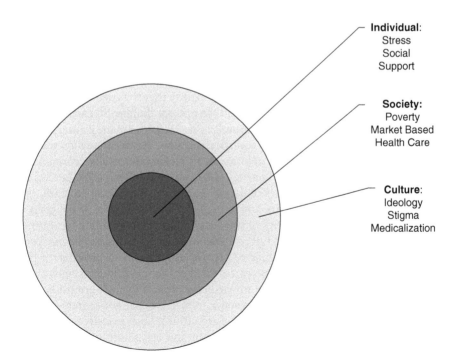

Individual:
Stress
Social
Support

Society:
Poverty
Market Based
Health Care

Culture:
Ideology
Stigma
Medicalization

Figure 7.1 Wholistic Framework for HIV Care and Research

organization of care), and macro (cultural beliefs and economic forces) influence and reinforce one another, and can help direct researchers to the ultimate sources of health care disparities.

The framework is also useful for community-based advocacy efforts, which need to move beyond market-based models of patient choice and consumerism to true democratic deliberation (Grob & Schlesinger, 2011). The major obstacles to patient empowerment described by Grob and Schlesinger (2011) target cultural and system-level barriers to social change, which I would identify as overarching social inequalities: a medicalized, individualized approach to disease, and a concern with technocratic rationality that emphasizes clinical efficacy and cost effectiveness rather than system-wide improvement. One of the reasons major efforts to integrate diverse systems of care have not been found to be efficacious or effective is outcomes are measured at the patient level (cost savings or quality of life), rather than at the system or even organizational level. Surely, an important measure of system integration is providers' knowledge of who to refer their clients to when faced with co-morbidities. Can we really expect major improvements to client-level functioning and quality of life when assessing the impact of long-term, chronic care diseases with no realistic hope of cure? Quite simply, no: This is why the only valid measures of both system-level integration and patient advocacy efforts have to be made in terms of processes. Are consumers and providers working to improve the system of care? It doesn't matter if these efforts are ultimately successful (Epstein, 2011), what matters is that people are working to change the rules of the game and to enhance the sense of the public good and collective patient identity (Grob & Schlesinger, 2011).

Ultimately, we need to move beyond the individual level to more complex understandings of systems of care if they are ever to be "wholistic" systems. Furthermore, we will have to confront the reality that the current system has been developed and is organized around the precept that health care is a commodity, and that profits and the accumulation of wealth are the primary goals motivating key stakeholders who control the system. Rather than incremental reform, our health care non-system needs to be fundamentally reorganized around a different goal—not efficiency (i.e., cost), but effectiveness (access to and quality of care). The values of quality care, or greater access to care, are goals that health care providers and patients have control over, while corporate forces push for the priority of the accumulation of wealth. The contradiction between providing the full continuum of care needed by chronic care populations and a system designed to provide as little care as possible (or the minimal amount of care that one can afford) is becoming increasingly obvious. The 2000 and 2001 Institute of Medicine reports identify contradictory principles for quality care: effectiveness, efficiency, patient-centered, safe, timely, and equitable (Timmermans & Berg, 2003). Each priority is also subject to processes of subjective interpretation and redefinition, with notable variations in what counts for effective treatment. For example, we now have efficient standards for effective mental health treatment—provided patients meet clearly defined DSM diagnostic criteria. Likewise, HIV and substance abuse also have their own standards of care.

While the needs of individuals with HIV disease, mental health, and substance abuse problems are diverse and met within different systems of care; in fact, this is one distinct population. Rather than being simply co-morbid (i.e., individuals with multiple conditions), HIV, MH, and SA operate synergistically. In addition, each separate condition is highly stigmatizing, and combined interactively, they produce unique barriers to care and treatment. Furthermore, many people living with HIV are disabled, and functional disability is also a consequence of prolonged mental health problems. Finally, a majority of individuals with HIV/MH/SA problems are racial minorities and indigent—adding to the outcast status of this particular group of individuals (Sontag, 1989). People living with HIV face daunting barriers to care and well-being; an adequate response to these obstacles has the potential to truly change the face of health care. If we can meet the challenges posed by this multiply disadvantaged group, we will be able to meet the challenges posed by increasing chronic health care problems among growing minority populations amid increasing levels of poverty. Currently, those studying chronic health care problems tend to focus on populations with relatively non-stigmatizing illness: old age, cancer, diabetes. These are common health problems known to afflict large segments of the population and are therefore not stigmatized. However, HIV, MH, and SA are highly stigmatized chronic care conditions, and there has been a lack of social commitment to provide adequate care or treatment.

Paul Farmer has written a great deal about our response to HIV and AIDS, and is also well known for linking his own advocacy efforts to larger issues of social justice, which is what I am attempting to do theoretically with the model depicted in Figure 7.1. Farmer (2005, pp. 152–153) argues that "the commodification of medicine invariably punishes the vulnerable . . . there is an enormous difference between seeing people as victims of innate shortcomings and seeing them as victims of structural violence." HIV disease, while a biological disease, is the result of social processes; it is embedded in unequal social structures, resulting in what Farmer (2005) refers to as structural violence. If we focus only on the individual and individual risk factors, either clinically or with our research, then the failure to provide access to HIV medications is reframed as non-compliance (Farmer, 2005). A focus on individual risk factors (or populations at risk) too often ends in blaming the victim (Farmer, 2005) and cultural stigma, which then serve as powerful obstacles to prevention and care. Likewise, with the rhetoric of cost containment, Farmer (2005, p. 177) agrees that excess costs must be curbed,

> but how can we glibly use terms like "cost effective" when we see how they are perverted into contemporary parlance? You want to help the poor? Then your projects must be "self-sustaining" or "cost effective" . . . the language of social justice is largely absent.

Community-based groups and advocates, as well as researchers, are forced in an environment of scarce resources (at least for HIV/AIDS, mental health, and substance abuse problems) to compete for funding to support research that cannot lead to any kind of significant changes to the system of care. But we must do more: We must work for what Farmer (2005) refers to as "preferential justice"—a system of care that sees the poor and disenfranchised as more, not less, deserving of care. We need to work to change the culture and social structures that surround the individual patient.

NOTES

1. The very success of the early HIV/AIDS patient advocacy movement by gay, White men led to later disputes over ownership of the disease and the social movement by women and people of color in the early 1990s (Epstein, 2011).
2. Epstein (2011) describes one obstacle to successful patient advocacy as conflict between different knowledge claims: those of the expert, or the expert-patient who have a good understanding of scientific knowledge, and those of the "lay-lay" activists, who based their knowledge claims in terms of their direct lived experience of a disease. In terms of my work with the HIV Council, I have often been challenged by "lay-lay" activists for not really understanding the HIV system of care as I am not a patient.
3. I use "holistic" to refer to integrated care at the individual or patient level, in keeping with medical literature, especially those in nursing. "Wholistic" refers to integration at the systems level, and is consistent with the use of that term in sociology.

Appendix A
Illness Narratives

How do you refer to your illness when you talk about it, or think about it?

What do you think your illness does? That is, how does it work?

How severe is your illness?

What kind of treatment do you think you should receive?

What are the important results you hope to receive from the treatment?

What are the chief problems the illness has caused?

What do you fear most about the illness?

What medications are you taking?

In what ways do these medications work?

What are some of the problems you have with these medications?

What are the things that you do to help with these problems?

Do you have anyone you can talk to about your problems with your illness or medications?

Who? Are they helpful? Why, why not?

Can you talk to any of your health care providers (e.g., your doctor, nurse, case manager, or pharmacist) about your problems?

If yes, who?

In thinking about your health care providers and the care that you receive, what things do you like best?

What do you like least?

In general, are your health providers and services available when you need them?

Do you have one health care provider with whom you have a fairly steady relationship?

How long have you known this person?

Is this a good relationship?

Appendix B
HIV/AIDS Adherence Tracking Forms

These forms have been developed by adherence counselors who have worked with clients on their adherence to HAART regimes during 2002 and 2003. While paperwork is always time-consuming, it is necessary to track referral, treatment planning, and adherence outcomes. Included in Appendix B you will find four forms:

1. Adherence Intake and Referral: This form will be completed when the client is first referred for adherence counseling. It can be completed by the referring health care provider, case manager, or adherence counselor.
2. Adherence Assessment Tool: This form will be completed when the adherence counselor first meets with a client to discuss adherence.
3. Adherence Treatment Planning: This is a tool for treatment planning and will be used on an ongoing basis.
4. Adherence Tracking: To be completed every 3 months to summarize treatment outcomes.

In order to help you keep track of adherence clients, we have found a tracking form to be useful. You can put this on your wall, calendar, or in your computer. You can quickly summarize the status of each client on this form (e.g., adherent, not yet on HAART, not adherent, drug holiday, etc.)

Client ID	Date of Initial Assessment	3 month	6 month	9 month	12 month

HIV/AIDS Adherence Program: Intake and Referral

Client ID: _____   Referral Date: _____

Emergency Contact:

_____

Referring Provider Name, Agency, and Phone Number:

_____

Other Service Providers (check if client is receiving services from):

Primary Care Physician/Clinic _____   ID Specialist/Clinic _____
Mental Health _____   Substance Abuse _____
Case Management _____
Current Pharmacy _____

Client HIV Status (check appropriate category):

HIV+ Asymptomatic _____   HIV+ Symptomatic _____
AIDS/CDC _____   Hepatitis C _____
Most recent viral load (give date): _____
Most recent CD4 count (give date): _____
Check Medications Client is on:

Class I: (NRTIS)	Class II: (NNRTIS)	Class III: Protease Inhibitors
___ Retrovir	___ Sustiva	___ Crixivan
___ Zerit	___ Viramune	___ Viracept
___ Videx	___ Rescriptor	___ Norvir
___ Hivid	___ Invirase	
___ Epivir	___ Fortovse	
___ Combivir	___ Agenerase	
___ Ziagen	___ Kaletra	
___ Trizivir		
___ Viread		

What other types of medications is the client taking (indicate specific health problem):

Reason for Adherence Referral:

_____ To Educate Client about HIV/AIDS
_____ To Educate Client about Proposed HAART Regime
_____ To Educate Client about Prescribed HAART Regime
_____ To Assess Adherence to Current Regime

Living Conditions of Client:

Own _____ Rent _____ Temporary/Emergency _____

With family/friends (stable) _____ With family/friends (unstable) _____

Homeless _____ Other (explain) _____

Substance Abuse? Yes _____ Maybe _____ No _____

Adherence Assessment Form (To Be Completed at Initial Intake)

Client ID: _____ Date: _____

What HIV medicines do you take?	How many times a day do you take this and when?	How many pills do you take with each dose?	Do you take it with or without food?

When was the last time you missed any of your anti-HIV pills?

1. _____ within the past week
2. _____ 1 to 2 weeks ago
3. _____ 2 to 4 weeks ago
4. _____ 1 to 3 months ago
5. _____ more than 3 months ago or never missed taking medications

Some people have problems taking HIV medications for various reasons. Have you missed taking your medications in the past 3 months because: (check all that apply)

1. _____ You have trouble remembering to take the pills at the right time?
2. _____ You get busy and forget to take your medications?
3. _____ You had too many pills to take?
4. _____ You did not want others to notice you taking the medications?
5. _____ The pills remind you that you have HIV?
6. _____ You're afraid the HIV medications won't work for you?

7. _____ You don't feel sick?
8. _____ You slept through dose time?
9. _____ You had side effects from medications?
10. _____ You did not refill your prescription?
11. _____ You felt depressed or overwhelmed?
12. _____ You had problems taking pills at specific times, with meals, or on an empty stomach?

(If it has not been done, arrange for a time to go through Barriers to Treatment Checklist with the client.)

Have you had problems with side effects from the medication?

_____ No

_____ Yes—If yes, read through the list and circle all that apply:

1. Rash   2. Diarrhea   3. Loss of appetite   4. Feeling tired
5. Headache   6. Stomachache   7. Tingling in hands or feet
8. Nausea or vomiting   9. Nightmares   10. Other _____

Do you believe your HIV drugs are helping you?

_____ Yes   _____ No   _____ Not Sure

Is your schedule the same from day to day?

_____ the same everyday

_____ different on weekends

_____ different on the days I go to work or school

_____ rarely the same

Do you eat meals at regular times?

_____ no or rarely _____ sometimes _____ most of the time

Write time of day: Breakfast _____

Lunch _____

Dinner/Supper _____

How often are you willing to take pills every day?

_____ never

_____ once a day

_____ 2 or 3 times a day

_____ more than 3 times a day

What is the best time for you to take medications?_____

Do you drink alcohol?

_____ No   _____ Yes   If yes, how often/much_____

Have you ever cut back or stopped taking your medications without telling anyone?

_____ Yes   _____ No

NOTES:

Adherence Treatment Planning

CLIENT ID: _____   COUNSELOR: _____

	Problem/Need	Plan/Activities	Date Achieved
Knowledge of HAART and HIV			
Beliefs regarding HIV, meds, healing, spirituality			
Experience with taking pills, herbs, etc.			
Depression, anxiety. In treatment for mental illness.			
ETHOL, substance use, Current/past			
Supports. Family/close friend			
Living situation Privacy issues			
Treatment goals Health goals			
Housing, food, safety			
Financial Resources: ADAP, Medicaid//Insurance Self Pay			
Other potential barriers or resources			

Adherence Tracking (To be completed every 3 months)

Client ID: _____   Date _____   Clinic _____

Adherence Counselor: _____

Viral Load: _____   CD4 _____   Date of Lab Work _____

Number of Client Contacts in Past 3 Months:

1. Office _____   2. Home _____   3. Phone contact _____

Number of Appts. Client has Missed in Past 3 Months: _____

Client Status at Follow Up (date above):

1. Client has dropped out—no contact
2. Client is not showing up for appointments
3. Client reschedules appointments, but does eventually show up with reminder
4. Client is showing up for appointments, but is non-adherent to some degree with meds
5. Client is adherent with medications as evidenced by (circle all that apply):
   - Lab work
   - Self-report
   - Your clinical assessment

If you have concerns about adherence, please describe them:

6. Client is deceased (give date) _____
7. Client has moved out of treatment area _____

Medication Update: (circle correct category)

1. Not on HAART _____
2. On HAART—No change in meds _____
3. On HAART—Change in meds: What? _____

New Health Problems: _____

Medication Refill History (if available):

No Evidence _____ Meds Refilled as Prescribed _____

Meds Not Refilled as Prescribed _____

How often do you believe client misses doses?

Never _____ Occasionally _____ Weekly _____

Daily _____ Why? _____

Educated Client Regarding (check all that apply):

HIV _____ Labs _____ Immune System _____

Medications_____ Resistance_____ Nutrition_____

Discussed with Client (check all that apply):

Substance Abuse _____ Regimen _____ Stress _____

Resources for living/meds _____ Mental Status _____

Referrals Made (circle all that apply):

Case Manager_____ Doctor_____ Pharmacist_____

Patient Education _____ Mental Health _____

Substance Abuse _____

Next Visit Scheduled: Yes _____ No _____

Summary of Adherence Client Outcomes

Use the client tracking form (to be updated every 3 months and attached here) to keep a summary of your client outcomes. Complete the Date of

Initial Assessment when you have met with the client and filled out the assessment form (after taking a referral). If you do not complete an initial assessment (e.g., you only met with the client once), then you would not report the client on the tracking form. Also, keep track of how many clients are referred to you for counseling, even if you only meet with them once.

0. Client is not on HAART
1. Client has dropped out—no contact
2. Client is not showing up for appointments but has been in contact
3. Client reschedules appointments, but does eventually show up with reminder
4. Client is showing up for appointments, but is non-adherent to some degree with meds
5. Client is adherent with medications (can include generally adherent with only occasional relapses)
6. Client is deceased (give date) _____
7. Client has moved out of treatment area _____

(You can use the number or your own shorthand for what category a client falls into—just keep track of 3-month outcomes on the form on the following page.)

Categories 1 and 2 would point to Non-Adherence.

Categories 3 and 4 point to Continued Work on Adherence (it is your call if Client's adherence is improving, or regressing).

Category 5 is Adherent.

Client ID	Date of Initial Assessment	3 month	6 month	9 month	12 month	Discharge Date (note adherence status using categories above)	6 month follow up Status after DC
Example Ts0922572	Sept. 2003	Dec. 2003 – 3 (reschedules but shows up)	March 2004 – 4 (showing up, non-adherent)	June 2004 – 4 (same)	Sept 2004 – 5 (Generally adherent)		

Calculation of Summary Report:

Just total the 3-month outcomes for your clients (go with your most recent progress note—if report is due in October and you last updated the progress note in August, use August).

Number of New Referrals since last report: 1. _____

ACTIVE CASELOAD:

Number of Clients you completed an intake assessment on
(not just new clients, but current total caseload):   2. _____
Number of Clients you are seeing who are still not on HAART (0):
3. _____
Number of Clients who have died or moved (6 or 7):
4. _____
Subtract clients not on HAART, those who died, or moved from Active
Caseload (2) (subtract lines 3 and 4 from 2):   5. _____
Number of Clients who you have not seen since initial assessment
(1 or 2: Non-Adherent):   6. _____
Number of Clients being seen on a regular basis who you are working
with to improve adherence (3 or 4):   7. _____
Number of Clients being seen on a regular basis with improved adherence (5):   8. _____
Number of Clients for whom you cannot determine adherence (e.g.,
maybe you haven't seen them since intake, or maybe there is conflicting
evidence of adherence):   9. _____
Number of Clients discharged since last report: 10. _____

NOTE: These clients will be also be counted as part of your active
caseload—even if they never came for adherence counseling (part of % non-
adherent), or if they were completely adherent and discharged adherent
(part of % adherent).
    Discharged Adherent _____   Discharged Non-Adherent _____

REPORT SUMMARY:

A. Percent of Active Caseload Non-Adherent: _____
(Calculate percentages by dividing line 6 by line 5 for total Non-Adherent)
B. Percent of Active Caseload Working to Improve Adherence: _____
(Add lines 9 and 7, divide total by line 5 for working to improve adherence:
Line 9 + Line 7 = _____ / Line 5)
C. Percent of Active Caseload Adherent: _____
(Divide line 8 by line 5 for improved adherence—total adherent/total
active caseload)

NOTE: The three percentages should total to 100.

COMMENTS:
What's working to improve adherence?
What problems are you encountering?

Appendix C
Integration Plan

OVERALL OBJECTIVES

To treat and educate as many HIV/SA/MH clients as quickly as possible through a client-centered, holistic approach. The current system of cooperation will move toward a more integrated state that combines:

1. an interagency coordinating body for HIV/SA/MH cases;
2. a multi-agency, multidisciplinary case management team;
3. cross-training of professionals and volunteers;
4. culturally appropriate and sensitive materials; and
5. preventative education and assertive outreach by paraprofessionals and community advocates to targeted minority populations at risk for HIV/AIDS.

Objective 1: Develop an interagency coordinating body for HIV/SA/MH cases.

Strategy:

Develop a group of provider and consumer representatives (at the local level) who are brought together to address common concerns. Their purpose will be to exchange information, needs assessment, identify areas for system coordination, and to promote access to comprehensive services. They will monitor the system to ensure that the overall mission is being met (this is the current EAB). In addition to the existing EAB, a coordinator position will be created and staffed. The coordinator will be responsible for coordinating the development of service contracts and joint proposals, providing overall assistance for implementing systems integration, ensuring that culturally appropriate and sensitive materials are available, monitoring cultural competence, organizing teams of paraprofessionals and community advocates to engage in assertive community outreach, and for developing and maintaining a community resource directory (see Objective 3). The coordinator will also oversee the multi-agency, multidisciplinary case management team.

Objective 2: Develop a multi-agency, multidisciplinary triage team that will be cross-trained and will assist agencies serving minority clients with cross-disability treatment needs.

The triage team will be comprised of professionals and consumers who have been cross-trained at all levels and who will build care maps. This team will develop common concepts and standards of care that address co-occurring illnesses and cross-cultural considerations. The team will develop, and modify as necessary, common screening and assessment tools to screen and treat clients with co-occurring illnesses. These instruments will also collect information on both formal and informal systems of care that will allow for a client-centered, holistic care plan.

Objective 3: Expand provider education of cross-disability and cross-cultural issues, and make cross-training system-wide.

Design and provide training modules for Level I, Level II, and Level III cross-training (See Chapter 5 in this volume).

Get credentialing authority for cross-training.

Provide training to implement common screening tools.

Develop a tool to assess level of skills and competencies of providers and direct care personnel (including volunteers).

Include volunteers, consumers, and consumer advocates in all levels of training, as appropriate.

Develop a community resource directory that will include information on the services offered by all agencies in the system, and will also list cultural partners in the community.

Objectives 4 and 5: Having developed a comprehensive system of care that is culturally accessible and able to meet the multiple needs of clients with co-occurring illnesses, there will be assertive community outreach to populations not currently receiving services. Targeted populations will be educated in culturally sensitive formats.

Teams of paraprofessionals and community advocates will engage in assertive community outreach to educate consumers and potential consumers, reduce barriers to care, improve access to services, and improve sense of trust in medical services. The teams will work with identified partners within the following targeted populations: (a) Black men, 18–25, non-gay identified who have sex with men; (b) women who have sex with previously identified population; (c) substance abusers; (d) populations engaged in sex for money or drugs; and (e) significant immigrant and minority populations.

Appendix D
Proclamation of December 1 as World AIDS Day (2012)

WHEREAS, AIDS and HIV have a global impact, with an estimated 33 million people living with HIV/AIDS and 25 million who have died worldwide; and

WHEREAS, an estimated 1.2 million Americans are living with HIV, and yet one out of five are not aware of their status; and

WHEREAS, North Carolina has reported 26,168 total AIDS cases from the beginning of the epidemic and North Carolina has ranked tenth highest among the 50 states in cumulative reported AIDS cases.

WHEREAS, HIV/AIDS continues to be a major health concern in Mecklenburg County, a community that includes over 5,000 people living with HIV/AIDS and an estimated one new case each day; and

WHEREAS, there is an increasing number of people at risk for HIV/AIDS in Mecklenburg County; and

WHEREAS, all citizens of Mecklenburg County living with HIV/AIDS deserve the right to adequate care, treatment, and services; and

WHEREAS, the epidemic of HIV/AIDS calls for national, state, and local efforts to prevent the spread of HIV/AIDS; and

WHEREAS, recognizing that continued commitments to combat HIV/AIDS are needed from all sectors of society, including families, communities, organizations, governments, and policy makers;

NOW, THEREFORE, BE IT RESOLVED that in conjunction with the global observance of World AIDS Day 2012, with the theme "Getting to Zero," the Mecklenburg Board of County Commissioners does hereby proclaim December 1, 2012 as

"WORLD AIDS DAY"

in Mecklenburg County and urges all citizens to take this day to remember individuals and their families who have been impacted by HIV/AIDS and to support people living with HIV/AIDS and to assist those who are in the fight to stop this epidemic.

References

Abbott, A. (1992). Professional Work. In Y. Hasenfeld (Ed.), *Human services as complex organizations* (pp. 145–162). Newbury Park, CA: Sage.

Abbott, A. (1988). *The system of professions: An essay on the division of expert labor.* Chicago: University of Chicago Press.

Alfonso, V., Geller, J., Bermbach, N., Drummond, A., & Montaner, J. (2006). Becoming a "treatment success": What helps and hinders patients from achieving and sustaining undetectable viral loads. *AIDS Patient Care, 20,* 326–334.

Altman, D., & Buse, K. (2014). *Thinking politically about HIV.* New York: Routledge, Taylor and Francis Group.

Andersen, R. (2000). Access of Vulnerable Groups to Antiretroviral Therapy among Persons in Care for HIV Disease in the United States. *Health Services Research, 35*(2), 389–466.

Anderson, G., & Knickman, J. R. (2001). Changing the chronic care system to meet people's needs: people with special medical and supportive care needs often have to navigate several disparate financing and delivery systems to obtain the services they need. *Health Affairs, 20*(6), 146–160.

Barfod, T. S., Sorensen, H. T., Nielsen, H., Rodkjaer, L., & Obel, N. (2006). "Simply forgot" is the most frequently stated reason for missed doses of HAART. *HIV Medicine, 7, 5,* 285–90.

Batki, S. L. (1990). Substance abuse and AIDS: The need for mental health services. *New Directions for Mental Health Services, 48,* 55–67.

Baumgartner, L. M. (2007). The incorporation of the HIV/AIDS identity into the self over time. *Qualitative Health Research, 17, 7,* 919–31.

Bauermeister, J. A., Tross, S., & Ehrhardt, A. A. (2009). A Review of HIV/AIDS System-Level Interventions. *AIDS & Behavior, 13*(3), 430–448. doi:10.1007/s10461-008-9379-z

Behavioral Social Science and Prevention Research Area Review Panel. Findings and Recommendations. (1996). *National Institute of Health AIDS Research Program Evaluation.* Washington, DC: Office of AIDS Research.

Benner, P. E. (1984). *From novice to expert: Excellence and power in clinical nursing practice.* Menlo Park, CA: Addison-Wesley Publishing Co.

Berger-Greenstein, J. A., Cuevas, C. A., Brady, S. M., Trezza, G., Richardson, M. A., & Keane, T. M. (2007). Major depression in patients with HIV/AIDS and substance abuse. *AIDS Patient Care & STDs, 21*(12), 942–955.

Bhatia, R., Hartman, C., Kallen, M., Graham, J., & Giordano, T. (2011). Persons newly diagnosed with HIV infection are at high risk for depression and poor linkage to care: Results from the Steps Study. *AIDS & Behavior, 15*(6), 1161–1170. doi:10.1007/s10461-010-9778-9

Bowleg, L. (2012). The problem with the phrase women and minorities: Intersectionality—An important theoretical framework for Public Health. *American Journal of Public Health, 102*, 7, 1267–1273.

Broadhead, R. S., Heckathorn, D. D., Altice, F. L., Van Hulst, Y., Carbone, M., Friedland, G. H., . . . Selwyn, P. A. (2002). Increasing drug users' adherence to HIV treatment: results of a peer-driven intervention feasibility study. *Social Science & Medicine, 55*(2), 235–246.

Brook, M. G., Dale, A., Tomlinson, D., Waterworth, C., Daniels, D., & Forster, G. (2001). Adherence to highly active antiretroviral therapy in the real world: experience of twelve English HIV units. *AIDS Patient Care & STDs, 15*(9), 491–494.

Burgoyne, R., & Renwick, R. (2004). Social support and quality of life over time among adults living with HIV in the HAART era. *Social Science & Medicine, 58*, 1353–1366. doi:10.1016/s0277-9536(03)00314-9

Burton, D. L., Cox, A. J., & Fleisher-Bond, M. (2001). *Cross training for dual disorders: A comprehensive guide to co-occurring substance use and psychiatric disorders.* New York: Vintage Press.

Butterfoss, F. D., and Kegler, M. E. (2012). A coalition model for community action. In M. Minkler (Ed.), *Community organizing and community building for health and welfare* (pp. 309–328). Rutgers, NJ: Rutgers University Press.

Cantor, J. A. (1995). Experiential learning in higher education: Linking classroom and community. ASHE-ERIC Higher Education Report No. 7. Washington, D.C.: The George Washington University: Graduate School of Education and Human Development.

Capece, M., & Schantz, D. (2000). An Approach to Community Facilitation Using Mediation Techniques: Skills for the Sociological Practitioner. *Sociological Practice: A Journal of Clinical and Applied Sociology, 2*(1), 23–32.

Carey, M. P., Weinhardt, L. S., & Carey, K. B. (1995). Prevalence of infection with HIV among the seriously mentally ill: Review of research and implications for practice. *Professional Psychology: Research and Practice, 26*(3), 262–268. doi:10.1037/0735-7028.26.3.262

Catz, S. L., Kelly, J. A., Bogart, L. M., Benotsch, E. G., & McAuliffe, T. L. (2000). Patterns, correlates, and barriers to medication adherence among persons prescribed new treatments for HIV disease. *Health Psychology, 19*(2), 124–133. doi:10.1037/0278-6133.19.2.124

Centers for Disease Control and Prevention. (2012a). Estimated HIV incidence among adults and adolescents in the United States, 2007–2010. HIV Surveillance Supplemental Report 2012, 17 (4). Retrieved from www.cdc.gov/hiv/topics/surveillance/resources/reports/index.htm#supplemtnal.

Centers for Disease Control and Prevention. (2012b). HIV in the United States: At a glance. Retrieved from www.cdc.gov/hiv/resources/factsheets/PDF/HIV_at_a_glance.pdf.

Center for Substance Abuse Treatment. (1998). Comprehensive Case Management for Substance Abuse Treatment. Treatment Improvement Protocol (TIP) series, Number 27. DHHS Pub. No. (SMA) 98-3222. Rockville, MD: Substance Abuse and Mental Health Services Administration, and Center for Mental Health Services.

Center for Substance Abuse Treatment. (2000). Substance Abuse Treatment for Persons with HIV/AIDS. Treatment Improvement Protocol (TIP) Series, Number 27. DHHS Pub. No (SMA) 00-314. Rockville, MD: Substance Abuse and Mental Health Services Administration, and Center for Mental Health Services.

Center for Substance Abuse Treatment. (2007). Services Integration. COCE Overview Paper 6. DHHS Publication NO. (SMA) 07-4295. Rockville, MD: Substance Abuse and Mental Health Services Administration, and Center for Mental Health Services.

Charmaz, K. (1991). *Good days, Bad days: The self in chronic illness and time.* Rutgers, NJ: Rutgers University Press.

Charns, M. P. (1997). Organizational Design of Integrated Delivery Systems. *Hospital Health Services Administration, 42*(3), 411–432.

Chernesky, R. H., & Grube, B. (1999). HIV/AIDS case management: views from the frontline. *Care Management Journal, 1*(1), 19–28.

Clay, S., Schell, B., Corrigan, R. W. and Ralph, R. O. (Eds.). (2005). *On our own together: Peer programs for people with mental illness.* Nashville, TN: Vanderbilt University Press.

Cohen, M. A. (1998). Emerging trends in the finance and delivery of long-term care: public and private opportunities and challenges. *The Gerontologist, 38*(1), 80–89.

Conover, C. J., Arno, P., Weaver, M., Ang, A., & Ettner, S. L. (2006). Income and Employment of People Living with Combined HIV/AIDS, Chronic Mental Illness, and Substance Abuse Disorders. *Journal of Mental Health Policy and Economics, 9*(2), 71–86. Retrieved from www.icmpe.org/test1/journal/journal.htm.

Conover, C. J., Weaver, M., Ang, A., Arno, P., Flynn, P. M., & Ettner, S. L. (2009). Costs of care for people living with combined HIV/AIDS, chronic mental illness, and substance abuse disorders. *AIDS Care, 21*(12), 1547–1559. doi:10.1080/09540120902923006

Conover, C. J., Weaver, M., Arno, P., Ang, A., & Ettner, S. L. (2010). Insurance coverage among people living with combined HIV/AIDS, chronic mental illness, and substance abuse disorders. *Journal of Health Care for the Poor & Underserved, 21*(3), 1006–1030. doi:10.1353/hpu.0.0330

Conrad, P. (2007). *The medicalization of society: On the transformation of human conditions into treatable disorder.* Baltimore, MD: John Hopkins University Press.

Cook, J. A., Cohen, M. H., Burke, J., Grey, D., Anastos, K., Kirstein, L., & Young, M. (2002). Effects of depressive symptoms and mental health quality of life on use of highly active antiretroviral therapy among HIV-seropositive women. *Journal Of Acquired Immune Deficiency Syndromes* (1999), *30*(4), 401–409.

Crystal, S., & Schlosser, L. R. (1999).The HIV-Mental health challenge. In A. V. Horwitz & T. L. Scheid (Eds.), *A handbook for the study of mental health* (pp. 526–549). Cambridge: Cambridge University Press.

Cunningham, C. O., Sanchez, J. P., Li, X., Heller, D., & Sohler, N. L (2008). Medical and support service utilization in a medical program targeting marginalized HIV-infected individuals. *Journal of Health Care for the Poor and Uninsured, 19*(3), 981–990.

Cunningham, W. E., Wong, M., & Hays, R. D. (2008). Case Management and Health-Related Quality of Life Outcomes in a National Sample of Persons with HIV/AIDS. *Journal of National Medical Association, 100*(7), 840–848.

Demmer, C. (2003). Treatment adherence among clients in AIDS service organizations. *Journal of HIV/AIDS & Social Services, 2*, 33–47.

Department of Health and Human Services. (2003). Guidelines for the use of antiretroviral agents in HIV-1-infected adults and adolescents. Retrieved from http://AIDSinfo.nih.gov.

Dill, A. P. (2001). *Managing to care: Case management and service system reform.* New York: Aldine de Gruyter.

DiPrete, T., & Eirich, G. (2006). Cumulative disadvantage as a mechanism for inequality: A review of theoretical and empirical developments. *Annual Review of Sociology, 32*, 271–297.

Earnshaw, V. A., Bogard, L. M., Dovidio, J. F., & Williams, D. R. (2013). Stigma and racial/ethnic HIV disparities: Moving toward resilience. *American Psychologist, 68*, 4, 225–236.

Eaton, W., Ritter, C., & Brown, D. (1990). Psychiatric epidemiology and psychiatric sociology: Influences on the recognition of bizarre behaviors as social problems.

In J. R. Greenley (Ed.), *Research in community mental health* (Vol. 6, pp. 41–68). Greenwich, CT: JAI Press.

Epstein, S. (1996). *Impure science: AIDS, activism, and the politics of knowledge.* Berkeley, CA: University of California Press.

Epstein, S. (2011). Measuring success: Scientific, institutional, and cultural effects of patient advocacy. In B. Hoffman, N. Tomes, R. Grob, & M. Schlesinger (Eds.), *Patients as policy actors* (pp. 255–277). New Overview paper 6 (Services Integration) and paper 7 (Systems Integration) are particularly useful and can be easily obtained from SAMHSA (www.coce.samhsa.gov)., NJ: Rutgers University Press.

Farmer, P. (2005). *Pathologies of power: Health, human rights, and the new war on the poor.* Berkeley, CA: University of California Press.

Farquhar, S. A., Michael, V. I., & Wiggens, N. (2005). Building on leadership and social capital to create change in 2 urban communities. *American Journal of Public Health, 94*(4), 596–601.

Fogerty, L., Roter, D. Larson, S. Burke, J. Gillespie, J., & Levy, R. (2002). Patient adherence to HIV medication regimes: A review of published and abstract reports. *Patient Education Counseling, 46*(2), 93–108.

Foster-Fishman, P. G., Salem, D. A., Allen, N. A., and Fahrbach, K. (2001). Facilitating interorganizational collaborations: The contributions of interorganizational alliances. *American Journal of Community Psychology, 29*(6), 875–905.

Freidson, E. (1984). The changing nature of professional control. *Annual Review of Sociology, 10*, 1–20.

Friedrichs, R. W. (1970). *A sociology of sociology.* New York: The Free Press.

Gentry, Q. (2007). *Black women's risk for HIV: Rough living.* Hawthorne, NY: Hawthorne Press.

Gielen, A. C., McDonnell, K. A., Wu, A. W., O'Campo, P., & Faden, R. (2001). Quality of life among women living with HIV: the importance violence, social support, and self care behaviors. *Social Science & Medicine, 52*(2), 315–322.

Goes, J. B., & Park, S. H. (1997). Interorganizational Links and Innovation: The Case of Hospital Services. *The Academy of Management Journal, 40*(3), 673–696.

Golin, C. E., Smith, S. R., & Reif, S. (2004). Adherence counseling practices of generalist and specialist physicians caring for people living with HIV/AIDS in North Carolina. *Journal of General Internal Medicine, 19*(1), 16–27. doi:10.1111/j.1525-1497.2004.21151.x

Grob, R., & Schlesinger, M. (2011). Principles for engaging patients in U.S. Health care and policy. In B. Hoffman, N. Tomes, R. Grob, & M. Schlesinger (Eds.), *Patients as policy actors* (pp. 278–292). New Brunswick, NJ: Rutgers University Press.

Harris, G. & Larson, D. (2007). HIV peer counseling and the development of hope: Perspectives from peer counselors and peer counseling recipients. *AIDS Patient Care and STDs, 21*(11), 843–860.

Hassett, S., & Austin, M. J. (1997). Service integration: Something old and something new. *Administration in Social Work, 21*, 9–12.

Health Resources and Services Administration. (2008.) CAREAction: Redefining Case Management. November 2008. US Department of Health and Human Services. Retrieved from hab.hrsa.gov-newspublications-careactionewsletter-november2008.pdf.0.

Hilfinger, M. D., Moneyham, L., Vyavaharkar, M., Murdaugh, C., & Phillips, K. (2009). Embodied work: Insider perspectives on the work of HIV/AIDS peer counselors. *Health Care for Women International, 30*(7), 572–594.

HIV/AIDS Treatment Adherence, Health Outcomes and Cost Study Group. (2004). The HIV/AIDS treatment adherence, health outcomes, and cost study: conceptual foundations and overview. *AIDS Care, 16*(sup1), 6–21. doi:10.1080/09540120412331315312

Hoffman, B., Tomes, N., Grob, R., & Schlesinger, M. (2011). *Patients as policy actors*. New Brunswick, NJ: Rutgers University Press.

Indyk, D., & Rier, D. A. (2006). Wiring the HIV/AIDS system: Building interorganizational infrastructure to link people, sites, and networks. *Social Work in Health Care, 42*(3–4), 29–45.

Institute of Medicine. (2001). Crossing the Quality Chasm: A New Health System for the 21st Century. Washington, DC.

Jia, H., Uphold, C. R., Wu, S., Reid, K., Findley, K., & Duncan, P. W. (2004). Health-related quality of life among men with HIV infection: effects of social support, coping, and depression. *AIDS Patient Care & STDs, 18*(10), 594–603.

Kaiser Family Foundation (2009). Ryan White and HIV/AIDS. Menlo, CA: Kaiser Family Foundation. Retrieved from KFF.org/hivaids.

Kaiser Family Foundation (2013a). The HIV/AIDS Epidemic in the United States. Retrieved from kff.org/hivaids/fact-sheet/the-hivaids-epidemic.

Kaiser Family Foundation (2013b). Medicaid and HIV/AIDS. Retrieved from kff. org/hivaids/Medicaid-and-hivaids.

Kalichman, S. C. Rompa, D., DiFonzo, K., Simpson, D., Austin, J., Luke, W., . . . Buckles, J. (2001). HIV treatment adherence in women living with HIV/AIDS: Research based on the Information-Motivation-Behavioral Skills model of health behavior. *Journal of the Association of AIDS Care, 12*(4), 58–67.

Kielmann, K., & Cataldo, F. (2010). Tracking the rise of the "expert patient" in evolving paradigms of HIV care. *AIDS Care, 22*, 21–28. doi:10.1080/0954012 1003721000

Kleinman, A. (1988). *The Illness Narratives: Suffering, Healing, and the Human Condition*. New York: Basics Books.

Klinkenberg, W. D., & Sacks, S. (2004). Mental disorders and drug abuse in persons living with HIV/AIDS. *AIDS Care, 16*(Suppl1), S22-S42. doi:10.1080/0954012 0412331315303

Knox, M. D. (1989). Community mental health's role in the AIDS crisis. *Community Mental Health Journal, 25*(3), 185–196.

Komiti, A., Judd, F., Grech, P., Mijch, A., Hoy, J., Williams, B., & Lloyd, J. H. (2003). Depression in people living with HIV/AIDS attending primary care and outpatient clinics. *Australian & New Zealand Journal of Psychiatry, 37*(1), 70–77.

Latkin, C. A., Donnell, D., Metzger, D., Sherman, S., Aramrattna, A., Davis-Vogel, A., . . . Celentano, D. D. (2009).The efficacy of network intervention to reduce HIV risk behaviors among drug users and risk partners in Chiang Mai, Thailand and Philadelphia. *Social Science and Medicine, 68*(4), 740–748.

Leutz, W. N. (1999). Five laws for integrating medical and social services: Lessons from the United States and the United Kingdom. *The Milbank Quarterly, 77*(1), 77–110.

Lichtenstein, B., Laska, M. K., & Clair, J. M. (2002). Chronic sorrow in the HIV-positive patient: issues of race, gender, and social support. *AIDS Patient Care & STDs, 16*(1), 27–38.

Light, D. (1997). The rhetoric and realities of community health care: The limits of countervailing powers to meet the health care needs of the twenty-first century. *Journal of Health Politics, Policy and Law, 22*, 106–145.

Link, B., & Phelan, J. (2001). Conceptualizing stigma. *Annual Review of Sociology, 27*, 363–385.

Longest, B. B. (1990). Inter-organizational linkages in the health sector. *Health Care Management Review, 15*, 17–28.

Lune, H. (2007). *Urban action networks: HIV/AIDS and community organizing in New York City*. Boulder, CO: Rowman and Littlefield.

Marquart, J. M., & Konrad, E. L. (1996). *Evaluating initiatives to integrate human services*. San Francisco: Jossey Bass Publishers.

McGuire J., Rosenheck, R., & Burnette, C. (2002). Expanding service delivery: Does it improve relationships among agencies serving homeless people with mental illness? *Administrative Policy in Mental Health, 29*, 243–256.

Mechanic, D. (1995). Sociological dimensions of illness behavior. *Social Science & Medicine, 41*(9), 1207–1216.

Mecklenburg County HIV Task Force. (2004). *Issues and recommendations for addressing HIV disease in Mecklenburg county.* A report to the County Commissioners.

Messias, D., Moneyham, L., Murdaugh, C., & Phillips, K. (2006). HIV/AIDS peer counselor's perspectives on intervention delivery formats. *Clinical Nursing Research, 15*(3), 177–196.

Meyerson, B., & Scofield, J. (1999). *Getting it together: State agency activity to coordinate substance abuse, mental health, and HIV prevention and treatment services.* Paper presented at the National HIV Prevention Conference.

Minkler, M., & Wallerstein, N. (2003). *Community-based participatory research for health.* San Francisco: Jossey Bass Publishers.

Mishler, E. (1989). Critical perspectives on the biomedical model. In P. Brown (Ed.), *Perspectives in Medical Sociology* (pp. 153–166). Belmont: Wadsworth.

Molassiotis, A., Lopez-Nahas, V., Chung, W. Y., & Lam, S. W. (2003). A pilot study of the effects of a behavioural intervention on treatment adherence in HIV-infected patients. *AIDS Care, 15*(1), 125–135. doi:10.1080/0954012021000039833

Molassiotis, A., Callaghan, P., Twinn, S. F., Lam. S. W., & Chung, W. Y. (2002). A pilot study of the effects of cognitive behavioral group therapy and peer support/counseling in decreasing psychological distress and improving quality of lie in Chinese patients with symptomatic HIV disease. *Aids Patient Care and STDs, 16*(2), 83–96.

Murphy, D. A., Marelich, W. D., Hoffman, D., & Steers, W. N. (2004). Predictors of antiretroviral adherence. *AIDS Care, 16*(4), 471–484.

Neugeboren, J. (1999). *Transforming madness.* Berkeley, CA: University of California Press.

Nnadi, C. U., Better, W., Tate, K., Herning, R. I., & Cadet, J. L. (2002). Contribution of substance abuse and HIV infection to psychiatric distress in an inner-city African-American population. *Journal of the National Medical Association, 94*(5), 336–343.

North Caroline Division of Public Health (2011). (2011). North Carolina HIV/STD Surveillance Report (2011). North Carolina Department of Health and Human Services, Communicable Disease Branch. Retrieved from http:epi.publichealth.nc.gov/cd/stds.

Parker, R., & Aggleton, R. (2003). HIV and AIDS related stigma and discrimination: A conceptual framework and implications for action. *Social Science and Medicine, 57*, 12–24.

Parsons, T. (1960). Structure and Process in Modern Societies. Glencoe, IL: The Free Press.

Pellowski, J. A., Kalichman, S. C., Matthews, K. A., & Adler, N. (2013). A pandemic of the poor: Social disadvantage and the U.S. HIV epidemic. *American Psychologist, 68*, 4, 197–209.

Pence, B. W., Gaynes, B. N., Whetton, K., Eron, J. J. Jr., Ryder, R. W., & Miller, W. C. (2005). Validation of a brief screening instrument for substance abuse and mental illness in HIV-positive patients. *Journal of Acquired Immune Deficiency Syndrome, 40*(4), 434–444.

Phillips, K. A., Mayer, M. L., & Aday, L. A. (2000). Barriers to care among racial/ethnic groups under managed care: ethnic minorities continue to encounter barriers to care in the current managed care-dominated U.S. health care system. *Health Affairs, 19*(4), 65–75.

Powell-Cope, G. M., White, J., Henkelman, E. J., & Turner, B. J. (2003). Qualitative and quantitative assessments of HAART adherence of substance-abusing women. *AIDS Care, 15*(2), 239–249.

Power, R., Koopman, C., Volk, J., Israelski, D. M., Stone, L., Chesney, M. A., & Spiegel, D. (2003). Social support, substance use, and denial in relationship to antiretroviral treatment adherence among HIV-infected persons. *AIDS Patient Care & STDs, 17*(5), 245–252.

Pradier, C., Bentz, L., Spire, B., Tourette-Turgis, C., Morin, M., Fuzibet, J. G., & Moatti, J. P. (2002). Adherence to therapy. Paper presented at the 9th Conference on Retroviruses and Opportunistic Infection, Session 73.

Prado, G., Lightfoot, M., & Brown, C. H. (2013). Macro-level approaches to HIV prevention among ethnic minority youth: State of the science, opportunities, and challenges. *American Psychologist, 68*, 4, 286–289.

Provan, K. G., & Sebastian, J. G. (1998). Networks within Networks: Service Link Overlap, Organizational Cliques, and Network Effectiveness. *The Academy of Management Journal, 41*(4), 453–463.

Pugh, G. L. (2009). Exploring HIV/AIDS case management and client quality of life. *Journal of HIV/AIDS & Social Services, 8*(2), 202–218.

Quander, L. (2000). HIV/AIDS and substance abuse: making connections with cross-training. *HIV Impact,* 1–2.

Raja, S., Teti, M., Knauz, R., Echenique, M., Capistrant, B., Rubinstein, S., . . . Glick, N. (2008). Implementing peer based interventions in clinic-based settings: Lessons from a multi-site HIV Prevention with Positives initiative. *Journal of HIV/AIDS and Social Services, 7*, 1, 7–26.

Reich, W. A., Lounsbury, D. W., Zaid-Muhammad, S., & Rapkin, B. D. (2010). Forms of social support and their relationships to mental health in HIV-positive persons. *Psychology, Health & Medicine, 15*(2), 135–145.

Reif, S., Smith, S. R., & Golin, C. E. (2003). Medication adherence practices of HIV/AIDS case managers: a statewide survey in North Carolina. *AIDS Patient Care & STDs, 17*(9), 471–481.

Relman, A. S. (1980). The new medical-industrial complex. *The New England Journal of Medicine, 303*(17), 963–970.

Rier, D. A., & Indyk, D. (2006). The rationale of interorganizational linkages to connect multiple sites of expertise, knowledge production, and knowledge transfer: an example from HIV/AIDS services for the inner city. *Social Work in Health Care, 42*(3/4), 9–27.

Roberts, K. (2000). Patient beliefs about antiretroviral adherence communication. *AIDS Patient Care & STDs, 14*(9), 477–455.

Rogers, C. R. (1969). *Freedom to Learn.* Columbus, OH: Merrill.

Rosenberg, C. (2007). *Our Present Complaint: American Medicine, Then and Now.* Baltimore, MD: Johns Hopkins University Press.

Ross-Friend, C., Schuster, A., & Sherry, M. (2011). Case management for people living with HIV/AIDS. *Care Management, 17*(3), 12–17.

Rubenstein, D., & Sorrentino, D. (2008). Psychotherapy with HIV/AIDS patients: Assessment and treatment plan development. *American Journal of Psychotherapy, 62*, 4, 365–375.

Safren, S. A., Otto, M. W., Worth, J. L., Salomon, E., Johnson, W., Mayer, K., & Boswell, S. (2001). Two strategies to increase adherence to HIV antiretroviral medication: Life-Steps and medication monitoring. *Behaviour Research and Therapy, 39*, 1151–1162. doi:10.1016/s0005-7967(00)00091-7

Scheid, T. L. (1994). An explication of treatment ideology among mental health care providers. *Sociology of Health & Illness, 16*(5), 668–693. doi:10.1111/1467-9566.ep11348763

Scheid, T. L. (2003). Managed Care and the Rationalization of Mental Health Services. *Journal of Health and Social Behavior, 44*(2), 142–161.

Scheid, T. L. (2004a). Service system integration: Panacea for chronic care populations? *Research in the Sociology of Health Care, 22*, 141–158.

Scheid, T. L. (2004b). *Tie a knot and hang on: Providing mental health care in a turbulent environment.* Hawthorne, NY: Aldine de Gruyter.

Scheid, T. L. (2007). Specialized adherence counselors can improve treatment adherence guidelines for specific treatment issues. *Journal of HIV/AIDS & Social Services, 6*(1–2), 121–138.

Schlesinger, M., & Mechanic, D. (1993). Challenges for managed competition from chronic illness. *Health Affairs, 12*, 123–137. doi:10.1377/hlthaff.12.suppl 1.123

Scott, R. W., Ruef, M., Mendel, P., & Caronna, C. A. (2000). *Institutional change and organizational transformation of the healthcare field.* Chicago: University of Chicago Press.

Shelton, R. C., Golin, C. E., Smith, S. R., Eng, E., & Kaplan, A. (2006). Role of the HIV/AIDS case manager: analysis of a case management adherence training and coordination program in North Carolina. *AIDS Patient Care & STDs, 20*(3), 193–204.

Shortell, S. M., Giles, R., & Anderson, D. (2000). *Remaking health care in America: The evolution of organized delivery systems* (2nd ed.). San Francisco: Jossey Bass.

Shortell, S., Zukoski, A. P., Alexander, J. A., Bazzoli, G. J., Conrad, D. A., Hasnain-Wynia, R. H., . . . Margolin, S. (2002). Evaluating partnerships for community health improvement: Tracking the footprints. *Journal of Health Politics, Policy and Law, 27*(1), 49–91.

Silver, E. J., Bauman, L. J., Camacho, S., & Hudis, J. (2003). Factors associated with psychological distress in urban mothers with late-stage HIV/AIDS. *AIDS & Behavior, 7*(4), 421–431.

Simoni, J. M., & Ng, M. T. (2000). Trauma, coping, and depression among women with HIV/AIDS in New York City. *AIDS Care, 12*(5), 567–580.

Smith, S. R., Golin, C. E., & Reif, S. (2004). Influence of time stress and other variables on counseling by pharmacists about antiretroviral medications. *American Journal of Health-System Pharmacy, 61*(11), 1120–1129.

Sontag, S. (1989). *Illness as metaphor and AIDS and its metaphors.* New York: Anchor Books.

Soto, T. A., Bell, J., & Pillen, M. B. (2004). Literature on integrated HIV care: a review. *AIDS Care, 16*, S43-S55. doi:10.1080/09540120412331315295

Stewart, K. E., Cianfrini, & Walker, J. F. (2005). Stress, social support and housing are related to health status among HIV-positive persons in the deep south of the United States. *AIDS Care, 17*(3), 350–358.

Stoff, D. M., Mitnick, L., & Kalichman, S. (2004). Research issues in the multiple diagnoses of HIV/AIDS, mental illness and substance abuse. *AIDS Care, 16*(Suppl1), S1-S5. doi:10.1080/09540120412331315321

Strauss, A. L. (1978). *Negotiations: Varieties contexts, processes, and social order.* San Francisco: Jossey Bass.

Strauss, A. L., Fagerhaugh, S., Suczek, B., & Wiener, C. (1985). *Social organization of medical work.* Chicago: University of Chicago Press.

Strauss, A. L., Schatzman, L., Burcher, R., Ehrlich, D., & Sabshin, M. (1964). *Psychiatric ideologies and institutions.* London: The Free Press, Jossey-Bass Publishers.

White House Office of National HIV AIDS Policy. (2010). National HIV/AIDS Strategy for the United States. Retrieved from http://aids.gov/federal-resources/national-hiv-aids-strategy/nhas.pdf.

Thoits, P. A. (2011). Mechanisms linking social ties and support to physical and mental health. *Journal of Health and Social Behavior, 52*, 2, 145–161.

Timmermans, S., & Berg, M. (2003). *The gold standard: the challenge of evidence-based medicine and standardization in health care*. Philadelphia: Temple University Press.

Tkatchenko-Schmidt, E., Atun, R., Wall, M., Tobi, P., Schmidt, J., & Renton, A. (2010). Why do health systems matter? Exploring links between health systems and HIV response: a case study from Russia. *Health Policy & Planning, 25*(4), 283–291. doi:10.1093/heapol/czq001

Trainor, A., & Ezer, H. (2000). Rebuilding life: The experience of AIDS after facing imminent death. *Qualitative health research, 10, 5,* 646–660.

Tsao, J. C., Dobalian, A., & Stein, J. A. (2005). Illness burden mediates the relationship between pain and illicit drug use in persons living with HIV. *Pain, 119*(1–3), 124–132.

Tucker, J. S., Burnam, M. A., Sherbourne, C. D., Kung, F. Y., & Gifford, A. L. (2003). Substance use and mental health correlates of nonadherence to antiretroviral medications in a sample of patients with human immunodeficiency virus infection. *American Journal of Medicine, 114*(7), 573–580. doi:10.1016/s0002-9343(03)00093-7

Vladeck, B. C. (2001). You can't get there from here: Obstacles to improving care of the chronically ill. *Health Affairs, 20*(6), 175–179.

Wainberg, M. L., & Cournos, F. (2000). Adherence to treatment. *New Directions for Mental Health Services* (87), 85–93.

Walkup, J., Satriano, J., Hansell, S., & Olfson, M. (1998). Practices related to HIV risk assessment in general hospital psychiatric units in New York State. *Psychiatric Services, 49*(4), 529–530.

Weaver, M. R., Conover, C. J., Proescholdbell, R. J., Arno, P. S., Ang, A., Uldall, K. K., & Ettner, S. L. (2009). Cost-effectiveness Analysis of Integrated Care for People with HIV, Chronic Mental Illness and Substance Abuse Disorders. *Journal of Mental Health Policy & Economics, 12*(1), 33–46.

Whetten, K., Reif, S. S., Napravnik, S., Swartz, M. S., Theilman, N. M., Eron, J. J. Jr., . . . Soto, T. (2005). Substance abuse and symptoms of mental illness among HIV-positive persons in the Southeast. *Southern Medical Journal, 98*(1), 9–14.

Whetten-Goldstein, K., & Nguyen, T. Q. (2002). *You're the first one I've told: New faces of HIV in the South*. New Brunswick, NJ: Rutgers University Press.

Wholey, D. R., & Burns, L. R. (2000). Tides of change: The evolution of managed care in the United States. In D. E. Bird, P. Conrad, & A.M. Fremont (Eds.*), Handbook of Medical Sociology* (5th ed., pp. 217–237). Upper Saddle River, NJ: Prentice-Hall.

Winiarski, M. G., Greene, L. I., Miller, A. L., Palmer, N. B., Salcedo J., & Villanueva, M. (2005). Psychiatric diagnoses in a sample of HIV-infected people of color in methadone treatment. *Community Mental Health Journal, 41*(4), 379–391.

Wisniewski, A. B., Apel, S., Selnes, O. A., Nath, A., McArthur, J. C., & Dobs, A. S. (2005). Depressive symptoms, quality of life, and neuropsychological performance in HIV/AIDS: The impact of gender and injection drug use. *Journal of Neurovirology, 11*(2), 138–143.

Wright, E. R., & Shuff, J. I. (1995). Specifying the integration of mental health and primary health care services for people with HIV/AIDS: The Indiana integration of care project. *Social Networks, 17*(3–4), 319–340.

Wyatt, G. E., Gomez, C. A., Hamilton, A. B., Valencia-Garcia, D., Gant, L. M., & Graham, C. E. (2013). The intersection of gender and ethnicity in HIV risk, interventions, and prevention. *American Psychologist, 68, 4,* 247–260.

Index

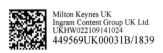